To my husband, thank you. A man's greatest gift to his wife is not to place her in subservience to him, manipulate or control her...but build her up, and edify her, so she can achieve all the plans God has for her. Thank you for being there for me in our ups, downs, in between, and supporting me while I have been growing through my healing and pain. I am thankful God provided me a safe place with you. You support me to Get Up, Be Raised Up, Grow. First Corinthians 13:4-8 says love is given in patience, kindness, without jealousy, or envy, in love that is not easily angered, protects, trusts, hopes, perseveres. I am strong now...and in God, I will not get lost. I appreciate sharing my journey with you as I learned to escape my Twisted Wonderland.

"But I don't want to go among mad people," Alice remarked. "Oh, you can't help that," said the Cat: "we're all mad here. I'm mad. You're mad."
Chapter 6, Pig and Pepper, Cheshire Cat and Alice

LEWIS CARROLL "ALICE'S ADVENTURES IN WONDERLAND" (1865).

CONTENTS

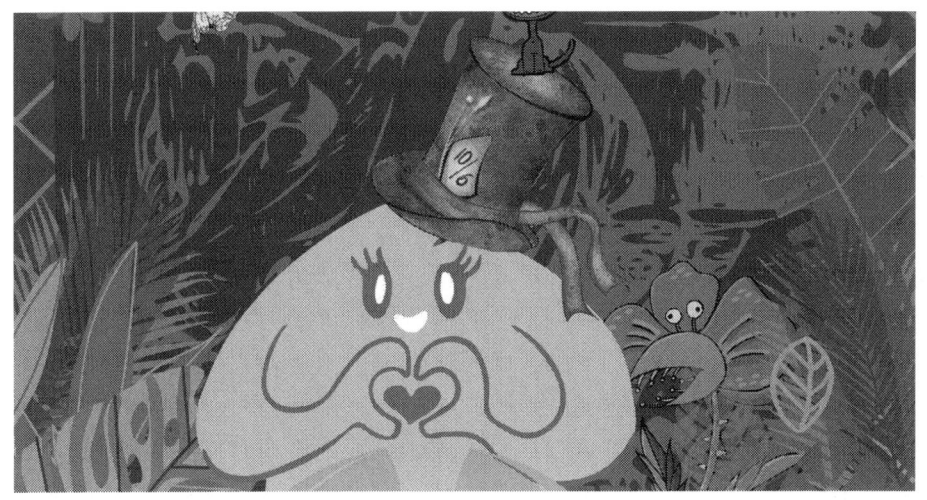

PROLOGUE

"Down, Down, Down, Fall I...Into the Rabbit Hole
It's hard to see my beauty through the pain
All I see are those very hard days.
The dead eyes staring back at me.
The silent scream echoing in my brain.
Where-ever have I gone, dear Alice?
Lost, confused, neglected, abandoned.
The day you left me in the parking lot...
Lost, scared, tired, confused, crying dying inside,
I did not know what to do.
It's hard to stay when my mind says go...
You calling me names I cannot always know;
What am I to answer to? Do I know?
What do I do but stay and take it?
In my heart I love you and leaving means breaking it.

What do I do when the tears won't dry?
When I cry out Father God, PLEASE help me when I want to die.
Heartbroken and lost I feel like I am alone.
Just like that little girl who felt the cold hard stone...
Every time that HE hit me all I could do was stay...
My days were so dark I lost my way."

(Chapter One Down The Rabbit Hole, *My Heart My Broken Heart*,
Buchanan, T., 2022).

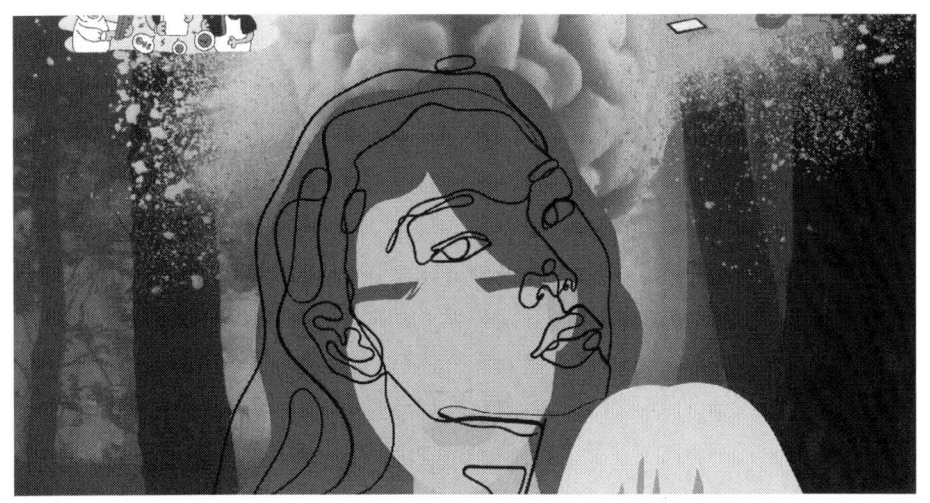

PREFACE

My Heart My Broken Heart books are a poem for this companion guide I wrote as a reflection of my thoughts and how I, in turn communicate empathy using metaphors and teachings in counseling to clients that enable them to feel validated in finally having a voice as we move through the process and various complex stages of healing. You are welcome to use the books (adult versions and child versions) for yourself, for clients if you are a clinician, share with a friend, reading group, or classroom. This guide is created to use WITH "My Heart My Broken Heart" stories, and may not seem to make sense to readers without the counterparts. It may read a bit *'mad'* and unorganized (like the neural network) should you use this guide alone; however, you may.

Unlike Lewis Carroll's Alice in Wonderland, characters used in my versions are not rational or reasonable. This guide conveys the irrational aspect of the damage to the brain in relational trauma. In examining my own *'madness'* of feeling shame and confusion, I share with you a semblance of ways you *may* feel about what has happened to you in your own emotional and psychological trauma of abuse. 'We can set to work,' and 'finish off the cake' without getting in the way and 'expecting nothing but out of the way things to happen' (a metaphor from Lewis Carroll's Alice's Adventures in Wonderland, 1865) for healing.

My Heart: My Broken Heart series includes an adult and children's version, journal books, and this companion guide to examine diverse aspects of *'madness'* of emotional and psychological abuse and based on characters of Lewis Carroll's *"Alice's Adventures in Wonderland,"* (Carroll, L., 1865) series. The various illustrations throughout 'My Heart My Broken Heart' series books are a plethora of mixed media from both Lewis Carroll (1865) originals I adapted and illustrated to match the emotional states within traumas of psychological physical and emotional abuse. *'My Heart My Broken Heart'* includes a collection of my original digital recreations and find and search and seek. My Heart My Broken Heart ADULT version includes aspects of feeling sexually used in young adulthood within romantic relationships.

This companion guide includes a *neutral* mixture of both versions with overall feelings and struggles Alice faces in the darkness of a dysfunctionally abusive twisted wonderland. This companion guide gives readers weapons to battle the war within our minds when we are feeling controlled by narcissistic abuser(s), and the mental toll is takes often stemming from childhood abuse.

Although I reference my own faith, and how I have been able to mentally grow strong, this book is not a *religious* book. This companion guide is a tool for ALL persons, no matter your personal belief systems. I revamped my original *"My Heart: My Broken Heart"* (Buchanan, 2022) for additional SPECIAL EDITIONS (hardback, paperback, E-Book) for adolescents to read and enjoy, for parents, clinicians, guidance counselors, leaders, mentors, and teachers to share with younger aged adolescents, along with journals for self exploration. This companion guide is an addition to those versions.

My Heart My Broken Heart Companion Guide book is my own exploration into the *'madness'* of the lostness of the psychological, physical, and emotional rabbit hole of abuse. It highlights effects of the mental toll of abuse from narcissistic parents or persons, and on oneself. I take you *all* into my dark twisted wonderland of feeling lost, trapped, manipulated, downtrodden, abused, neglected, rejected, abandoned, guilted, shamed, degraded. I take you with me into my past into the very darkest places of loneliness one finds oneself because of abuse.

This companion guide is an eye-opening experience for you to feel emotionally connected to students, mentee's, foster children, those whom you care for, including yourself, Dear Alice's. Let's journey together and come out of Time's loop of destruction and demise. Together, I can show you how to come out of your own Twisted Wonderland, and find the MUCHNESS that is you that has been hiding for far too long, *Real Alice.*

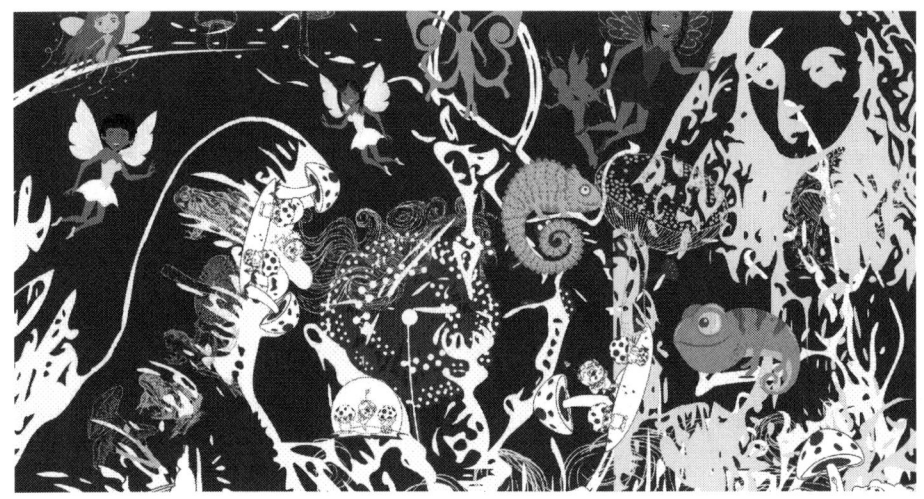

INTRODUCTION

I, like Alice, during childhood and young adulthood, found myself lost in a Twisted Wonderland, wondering in circles while my *'muchness'* got lost within. I experienced childhood behavioral issues, ongoing bullying, early complex chronic trauma, substance abuse in early teens, what *seemed* to present as oppositional defiance, and a plethora of issues with teachers who triggered me. I was named *"Trouble."* I failed most of my early education and coping was difficult.

I was traumatized and my safe persons and safe places were compromised at various intervals of *Time's* control. I had no healthy outlets in school such as sports because of my grades and undiagnosed mental health struggles. I was not offered counseling. Counseling was not something many people did. I was able to feel like 'me' around a select small group of individuals who I counted on to have my back...until Time's demise and destruction stepped in and I lost my muchness. I became Twisted Alice.

Unresolved chronic trauma kept me feeling as though I were trapped in a loop of destruction. I was moved from those I counted on to feel safe around and thrown into a twisted loop where I felt I had no control, no value, no power. I was lost in Twisted Wonderland for most of my teenage years and young adulthood. This compation to the 'My Heart My Broken Heart' books is dedicated to *all* Twisted Alice's, so you may learn there are others who may be experiencing abuse, neglect, bullying, suicidal thoughts, using actions of self-harm, using substances to escape, struggling with behavior issues because of tough stuff going on at home no one knows about...those who exhibit anxiety, depression, irritability with other peer group interactions...you name it within abusive destructive relationships.

I found my *muchness* in my adulthood where I learned to heal, focusing my strengths, and my pains into growing educationally. I learned to hone my strengths (stubbornness, tenacity, resilience) into counseling at Acorns n Bones OMC. I learned HOW to come out of Twisted Wonderland, and break the destructive loop *Time* had captured within my mind from early trauma. I found my MUCHNESS and decided to let it shine. I earned consistent *Summa cum laude* honors exceeding the plethora of unhealthy labels and boxes I was thrown into by others who were *"mad"* in my childhood and young adulthood. I learned to forgive (myself) and set healthy boundaries to forgive my abusers.

Professionally, I am Dr. Tia Buchanan, a Licensed Professional Counselor, LPC Supervisor, Licensed Addiction Counselor, NCCA Licensed Clinical Christian Counselor, NCCA Certified Sexual Therapist, EMDR Clinician, DCEMin., M.A., M.A, M.S., Certified Play Therapist, Court Involved Therapist, Certified Six-Sigma Black Belt. Since 2010, I have counseled families, teens, adults, and adolescents for a wide range of issues, depression, anxiety, ADHD, trauma, and focus most of my clinical and educational work on community care coordination and traumatology from a developmental psychology foundation.

My educational background includes *earned Summa cum laude* honors. I have earned an Associate of Applied Sciences Crim-

inal Justice: Criminology and Family Law; Bachelor of Theology; Master of Christian Counseling, NCCA Ordained Credentials as Licensed Clinical Christian Counselor; NCCA Licensed Advanced Board Certification Sexual Therapy; Master of Arts Human Services Marriage and Family Therapy Cognate, Master of Professional Counseling (CLINICAL); Doctorate Christian Ministry Counseling Education; Certification as a Six-Sigma Black Belt, Post-Master Certification Play Therapy,
Master of Applied Sciences Forensic Psychology: Mental Health Applications: Pediatrics.

I have conducted various Court Involved Therapy cases within scope and practice of legal aspects of custodial parent child attachment and reunification therapy within pediatrics. I educationally hold specializations in adolescent and adult personality disorders. Currently, I am undergoing a second Doctorate in Developmental Psychology with a minor in Education Community Care and Counseling: Traumatology. I am also an ISSA Certified Elite Personal Fitness Trainer, ISSA Certified Yoga Instructor, and ISSA Certified Kickboxing Instructor and Coach. I serve from a whole person bio-psycho-social-spiritual foundation.

As a Licensed Professional Counselor and clinician one mantra for me is continuous process improvement to provide *quality* care outside of the box of traditional therapy. Being competent in the ability to pull from a wide range of hats (sometimes *"we're all mad here"*). I treat individuals suffering from psychiatric illnesses, psychosomatic disorders and behavioral issues stemming from childhood physical, emotional, neglectful, sexual abuse, and trauma. Experiencing various life events may be negatively encoded into our memory bank and affect our bio-psycho-social-spiritual ability to process events adaptively to situations, persons, our environments, and affect our natural ability to recover from distressing events. Sometimes, we feel *mad* (angry mad, even rageful like an exploding volcano inside) and we may not know why.

I learned throughout my own journey from Twisted Wonderland, I had the power to make CHOICES for me, and I was not obligated to carry other peoples baggage, or their opinions of me because *they* wanted to control me through abusive narcisstic destruction. I learned to heal from childhood traumas, and recognize WHEN I was being targeted through manipulative abuse. I learned to *Get Up, Be Raised Up, Grow* OUT of Twisted Wonderland...and this guide is to teach you to do that for yourself too, Real Alice's, because the world needs you!

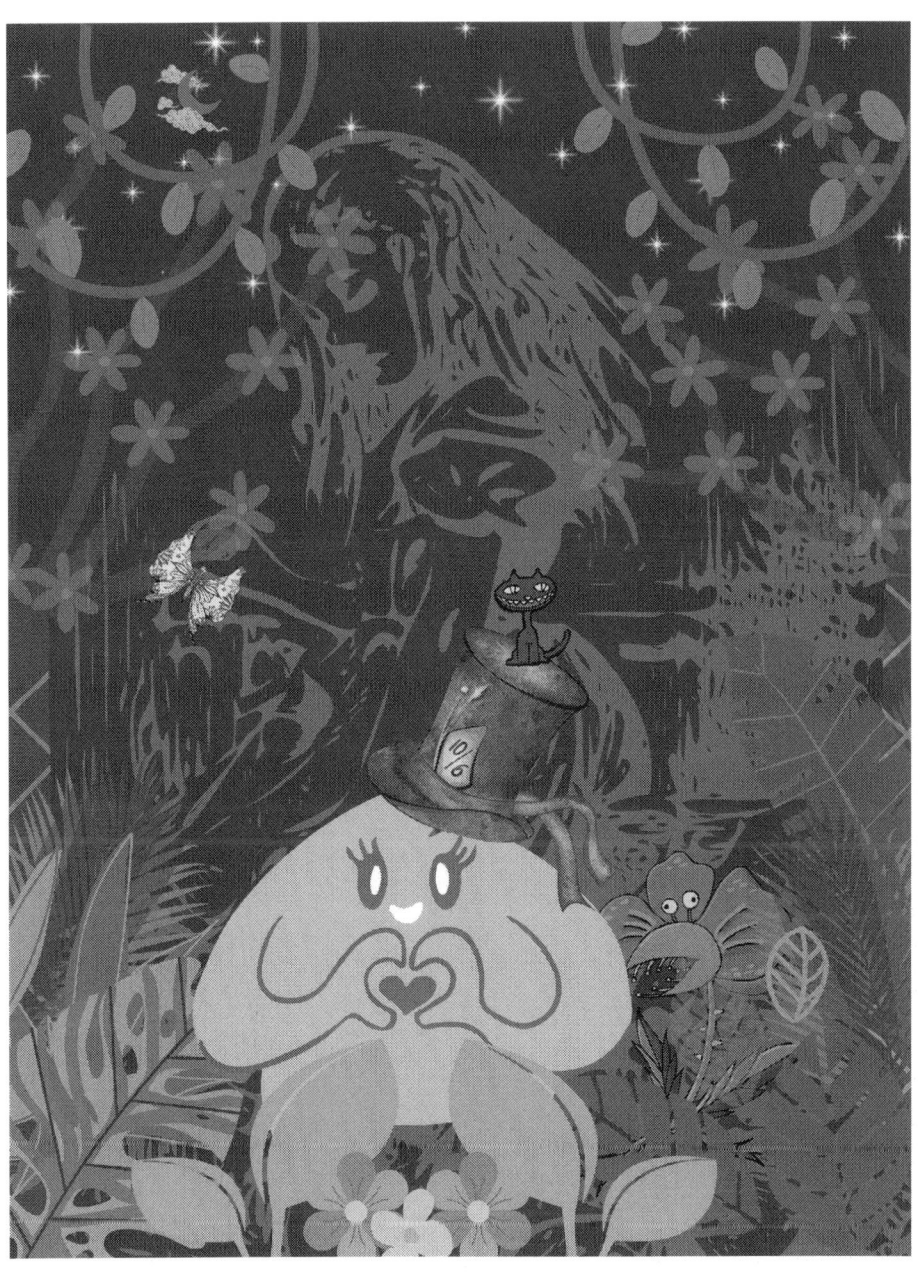

MY HEART MY BROKEN HEART COMPANION GUIDE

Dr. Tia Buchanan, M.A., M.A., M.S., DCMin., LPC, LPCS, LAC, NCCA, ISSA, EMDRC, CPT

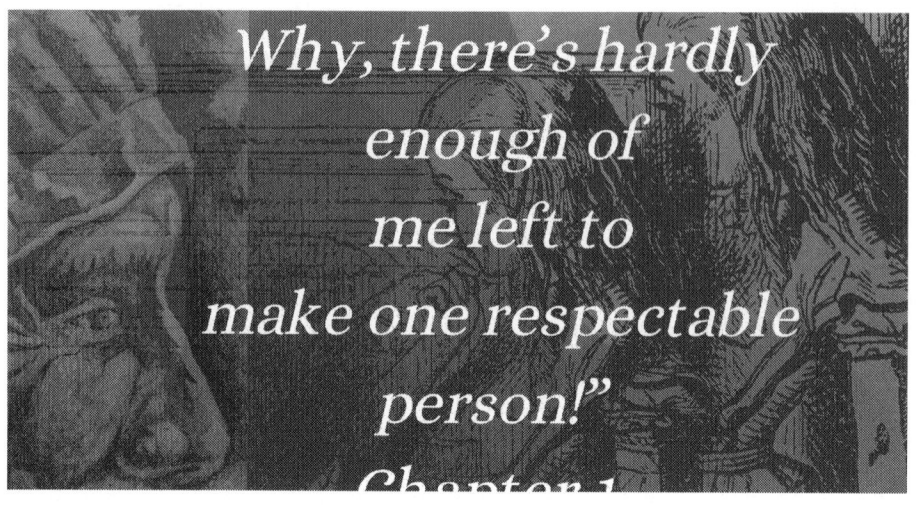

Why, there's hardly enough of me left to make one respectable person!"

Chapter 1

CHAPTER ONE

Down the Rabbit Hole

Trauma of a Twisted Wonderland

There are many tools' narcissistic abusers play in their games of control and dominance. Like chess, they use players to achieve one outcome: to *destroy* or *possess* the queen. Throughout this companion guide, I will show you HOW they seek to accomplish this successfully through *time*, as Time. You will learn how the brain becomes traumatized and stuck. I will teach you the various tools used by narcissistic abusers, how the tools are used, and how trauma affects you. For example, one tool is PR. A narcissistic abuser will use supporters to attack those who try to prove misdoings on the narcissist's part. These are *pawns.* They plan plot and play out the game of public relations (like an agent hired for an actor/actress who speaks only highly of the abuser and hides their destructiveness).

With a narcissistic abuser, you, Dear Alice's, will be blamed for whatever is *done* to you, and for how you respond when you buck their demeaning authority and control. Blame *will be* projected onto all persons in your support group, who dare to participate in revealing truth because accusations are how a narcissistic abuser will heap blame onto whoever else they can to take attention *off* themselves. (Smoke and mirrors, deflecting). As things continue to devolve, *their* lies increase and are repeated endlessly. They will paint themselves in the most glowing light, taking credit for things others have done and rewrite history to further support their perfection and superiority (and through PR). The goal is to control you through demise and destruction, Dear Alice's.

When you leave the relationship, the narcissist will go to any length to get you back into their life when he/she does not have supply (or PR gets too close to real rather than fakery). You may occasionally mistake trickery (and thier flattery) for genuine remorse and a desire to make things work (or for them to get short term therapy and help if you will just come back). This is a *calculated* appeal to your sentimentality and timed to catch you at a weak moment...most often when you feel vulnerable or reflective. This is a scheme *meant to toy with your emotions* to get you to soften up and reconcile.

The narcissist is a master at hiding personality and behavior abnormalities (and pathological agendas). Like the queen in *Lewis Carroll's* stories, you feel *mad*...only you are not mad (like a coocoo bird), Dear Alice, you have become *lost,* and that is exactly where they want you to be.

Healing From Twisted Wonderland

I had to heal from long term narcissist abuse. We all either choose to heal (present for future), or chose to remain Twisted (from the past). To you, my fellow *Queens* and *King's,* **Real Alice's,**

I SEE you. I hear your voices in the night. I reach out and I feel the strength waning, hear you struggling to swim in the sea of tears, and fight against the waves of the tenacity of deadened dark tendrils of despair you leak in your anguish and confusion. BUT FOR GOD stepping in for me, and healing me, I would have emotionally drown. In my own healing I am now able to sit patiently and empathically with every tear you cry from your own *madness* (pain) and in your own darkness. Your pain leaks into the atmosphere, and finds me even before I meet each of you. As an empath with the spiritual gift of prophesy, mercy, and discernment, I feel the intense anguish you are trapped within...and I do not absorb it into myself. Rather, I give to you a gift. As you pour yourself into healing while immersing yourself in this companion guide, I am praying for each of your hearts and minds for genuine healing. I am praying for you to find *your* way in your MUCHNESS.

Your pain finds me in your madness and that is *my* purpose, my gift, my strength. My muchness has been shared in the "My Heart My Broken Heart" series with you so you will *learn* to recognize, find, and accept *your* muchness and come out of the Twisted Wonderland of abuse. My abuse and pain provided a gift of healing for you to allow these words to come alongside you, *Dear Alice's*, and show you a way out of the nightmares of twisted wonderland and dark dismal roads of despair that narcissistic abusers have used to attempt to keep you trapped within.

It is hard to see 'your' beauty through the pain...and sometimes all we can see are those very hard days. To heal, *Dear Alice's* you are the ones who have to decide to choose your muchness through your own dark journeys of the never-ending cycle of empty hallways full of running numbers and nausea of traumatic triggers and memories from the ones who have abused you.

The choice to heal involves re-teaching healthy concepts, and re-wiring the brain in a professional setting with trauma recovery. It isn't easy by any means. Especially when you are manipulated to endure pain because of judgement, shame, guilt, condemnation, belittlement, others blaming you for their behaviors, stealing the joy you can no longer find within.

Professionally, I see many forms of Twisted Alice's...those who identify as Christian, non-Christian, LGBTQ2+, those who are of other religions, all demographics, all ages and *mostly* teens and young adults. I have clients tell me they were told by family members, parents, church families, leaders to '*overlook* abuse, to *forget* it because to forget for them falsely, means 'forgive'...just '*don't* talk about it,' '*dont* press charges,' and '*don't expose* the abuse' because '*you* will ruin them.' I hear from clients, they are told 'They are 'such great folks, you must have done...(something) to provoke or cause the abuse' or not to come forth because 'they are family' and 'it will be handled.' This is what abusers count on people saying, doing, and forcing onto others to believe

Narcissistic abusers use others for public relations (PR) (the people involved in protecting the abusers image in public at all costs). They use the tool I speak of later called gaslighting on behalf of the narcissistic abuser and are: (1) pawns being used, (2) narcissistic abusers themselves, and can be (3) VERY ignorant of the way God created our human brains to function within a biological psychological sociological and spiritual whole person foundation. (Regardless of status or class).

I love (*my*) church home...and I do not down 'church' as in a place to gather and praise God. What I do *not* give place to in examples clients share with me about PR of abusers is the use of pure evil, those who manipulate and abuse people, those who are ignorantly *purposely* used by evil to allow the begetting of generations of abusive physical psychological and sexual violations that create *long term chronic complex trauma*. Those who abuse religion to hide abuse...it is a disrespect to the character of God (many claim to serve) Who is loving. Narcissistic abusers use others *publicly* to gain power, control and for manipulative purposes to keep victims QUIET (at all costs). PR perpetuates abuse and covers up detrimental chronically long term pervasive pain and anguish all because someone is protecting the abuser. You learn to "shush be quiet stupid Alice! or he'll remember you girl!"

I have clients who have said they did not come to counseling for chronic relational trauma, or after getting out of abusive relationships because they were told to pray, smoke, or drink their pain away. (Depending on who was trying to 'help' them through it. The false collective that everything would be okay because we can merely 'forget' it does not work. Pretending it did not hurt does not work. The pain comes back because the brain responds to trauma differently than the narrative to just be quiet. Miracles and healing I *have seen* (I have healed!) AND I have also examined concepts of the processes of developmental brain structures in traumatology we will talk more about later too.

Trauma experienced during narcissistic abuse (and during childhood, specifically) *alters* the **entire structural development** of the corpus callosum, hippocampus, and amygdala. Although other brain regions are altered by trauma exposure, these *three* are the most deeply and adversely affected. (I will examine this in more detail with you in later chapters.) For now, we have been *created* for our brains to *encode* events. **Encoding** is the initial step in creating memories and is a *biological* phenomenon, rooted in our senses, and beginning with perception. We need to de-program abuse in order to heal from the time our minds were hijacked because events (including: people, senses, energy, negative self thoughts, judgments of others, abuse type, environment, support systems present or not present, critical self, critical parent/caregivers/lovers, child self, balanced lost self, what was done about the abuse, who hide it) is encoded into the file locked onto the path of our neural networks (pathways down dark rabbit holes).

The brain will throw us down into these maladaptively (negative) encoded rabbit holes out of nowhere of twisted wonderland where we are trapped in the time loop of these events. Meanwhile the narcissistic abuser (what they look like, smell like, what they did, how they hurt us) can be *so strong* within our memory bank system, the prefrontal cortex, hippocampus, and amygdala have been rewired and do not know HOW to unloop the destruction from within. Flashbacks and memory loss occur because grey matter shrinks in our brain! We grow and shrink and can no longer respond rationally.

In this companion guide, I will teach you more of how

the brain works in trauma...and why, although I affirm healing of hands and miracles God provides, also acknowledge He gifted people *(like me)* as therapist's for a reason. My gift is to help you traverse through deep waters filled with your own tears having fallen and gotten trapped in the darkness where the mind has many mansions, some filled and decorated with traumatic muck and mess we do not always want to visit, sit inside of, and often ignore, and do not know how to stop drowning in. The narcissistic abuser seems to have all of the power. We seem to feel lost, helpless, alone. While they PR their way into being seen as wonderful, we fall deeper into the darkness, alone.

The younger parts of us (any age before today is younger than you, happy un-birthday by the way), are trapped within those timelines of memories. Those little you's, Little Alice's are stuck in time *still* hurting, screaming, crying, dying inside in Twisted Wonderland. Those dark days and dark holes are very deep within the neural network. Sometimes the younger Twisted Alice's are trapped within shadowy holes of dysfunctional wonderland and are screaming to be heard, validated, assured, healed, reconciled, delivered. *They* want to see justice served...they want people to STOP listening to the abuser and stop seeing the abuser as such a goodie goodie! They want to stop hearing people PR for the abusers who protect the abuser!

These little you's are unique little parts of self that are leaking in thier anguish *because* they are trying to scream and yell their way out because they have fallen down, down, down so far. No one seems to hear them. They are invisible. They are unloved. They are devalued. They are unappreciated. They are abused.

In healing, to get to the *Real Alice*, you either choose *you* or the rabbit in the hole that grew into a jabberwocky trapped by Time (you can read about this in My Heart My Broken Heart editions), whom you followed into the darkness when curiosity led what your eyes thought thcy saw, what others *told* you to follow, to do, or because you were placed or born into the world of a twisted nightmare by a narcissistic abuser(s) who trapped you and held you captive.

Some days it seems normal to feel mad, and most days we try to forget. We use behaviors to cope with the darkness and we try to just feel good for once in the twistedness of depravity. Forgetting does not help us heal…and talking about it can sometimes re-traumatize. Meanwhile, the abuser looks great to the public.

Substances, sex, gambling, shopping, any addiction is a way to try and alleviate our pain, to forget the traumas intrusiveness into the *here and now*, and we just want to feel pleasure or pain to punish ourselves. Our brain is originally wired for pleasure, and when we hurt, we try to get that back. Alice said *"there is no use in crying like that…"* to herself, and rather sharply. She too, scolded herself much too harshly and severely. Often we feel like two different people because of the complexities of the narcissistic abuse. We do not know who to be…we can feel like ourselves one minute and confused and confuzzled the next.

The White Rabbit

There is hardly room for us to pretend to be two people because there is hardly room for one respectable person. We want to take what we see in the little glass boxes presented in front of us, and sometime disappear, sometimes shrink small, sometimes grow large to scare the narcissistic abuser away. Some days we just do not care what happens to us. We scream *which way*! Which way!

One minute we are being complimented by the narcissist and the next minute we are being accused and ridiculed. They are adapt at showing their Cheshire stripes at home where we see their true colors shining through…but in public, the mask is charming, manipulative, friendly, they have an audience, and are skillful at when and with whom they reveal themselves. We are the *queens* they set to destroy in their game of chess and others are their *pawns*…doing their public bidding.

Women (*and men*) are hesitant to admit to being narcissistically abused and may fail to obtain assistance to heal after (or during) an 'abusive' relationship. It takes time to label the duck a duck and call the relationship accurately *'abusive.'* That is part of the programming too you know...don't talk about it! And when you do, you must be *a liar* because the narcissist (and their PR) convinces everyone he or she is a goodie two shoes pillar of the community (White Rabbit's). *(John Wayne Gacy was also good at convincing others he was good.* That is what they naturally can do).

The situations and interactions with a narcissistic abuser can be frightening and confusing AND can also seem safe and secure *(at first)*. They will attempt to drag your support systems to them to use and manipulate you into *their* circle or align your support systems to *their* side by showing favor and feigning a false sense of security and attachment.

Narcissistic abusers are methodical planners and you must be ten steps ahead knowing and recognizing what their behaviors mean. They will use friends and family members close to you to convince them their behaviors were *'not really'* abusive or bad, or provocative or provoking to you...*you're* just overdramatizing.

One moment down went Alice after (the rabbit) down the hole, never once considering **how in the world** *she was to get out again...*

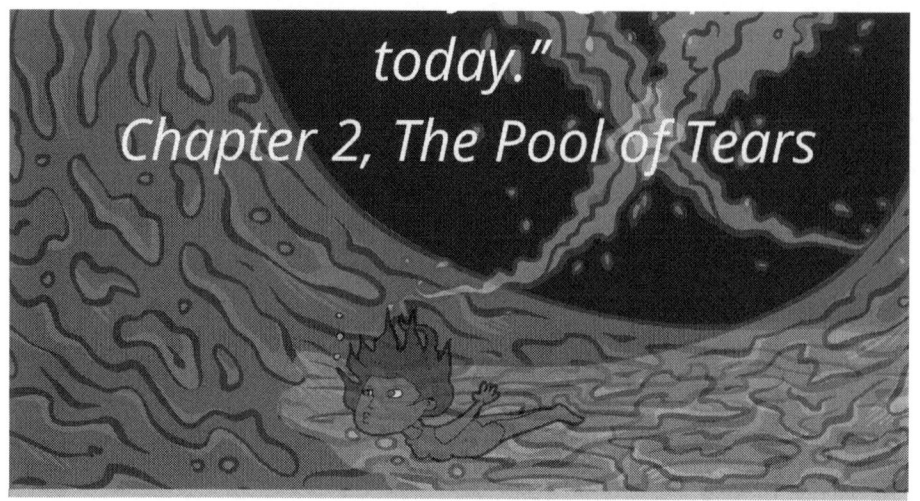

CHAPTER TWO

The Pool of Tears

Narcissistic abusers will focus on your shortcomings and judge you openly. They will do so in such a way others see you for those *perceived* shortcomings and even use your truths and secrets to achieve this goal. When you finally speak out about the (often) *years* of abuse you may find yourself doubting your reasons for your boundaries with a foundation of a false narrative from others to discount your experience with 'maybe it wasn't that bad,' 'he or she would never,' 'he or she is so nice!'

They NEED others to idolize their social identities! This gives them power to continue the cycle of shame and guilting you back into their circle of resources. They believe that whatever they need to do to get what they want is justified! You, Alice's, go through a rabbit hole straight through a long tunnel for such a way, dipping suddenly down, and you do not have a moment to think about yourself before you find yourself falling in a deep, very deep, well.

The myth *'Abuse doesn't happen to strong women'* is WRONG. Each of us has our own created unique temperament, changed by social roles, constraints, abuse, violence, cultural viewpoints of religious rules (that do not necessarily have a value or say-so from *Yahweh).* Domestic and narcissistic abuse (in childhood or adulthood) has no gender, color, class, health, or religion. You cannot get out as easily of a situation as others think...*your brain has been hijacked!*

Not all narcissistic abusers use substances such as alcohol or drugs. As children and adolescents, we cannot often leave an abuser's home. Up to 5% of persons have NPD (Narcissistic Personality Disorder). It appears in late teen and early adulthood. However, for some, the presentation stems from early childhood attachment disorders, and can be an issues in early adolescence and seen in other ways in adolescents with borderline personality, histrionic, antisocial disorders. As a pediatric developmental clinician, I do work with youth who are diagnosed with personality disorders as reflective of deviations from their stages of development. In adolescent stages, early interventions help mitigate the pervasive pattern of dysregulation when trauma and attachment work are part of their treatment plan. In adulthood, patterns often do not change...they merely hide for a time. They demonstrate neurocognitive deficits with a history of abuse that have altered their ability to regulate and feel genuine empathy for others.

Narcissistic abusers patterns do not change, and these patterns are not *situational* for them. It is about the synaptic programmed response to motor, emotional, and cognitive aspects of the brain. They manifest more in certain situations because they need control and power. This is a pervasive pattern, and deeply ingrained as distressful ways in thinking feeling and behaving. They have difficulties maintaining healthy relationships and bound-aries others need to have for themselves to be healthy due to their own self destructive tendencies and impairments. Common manifestations include manipulation, deceitfulness, destruction of others belongings, breaking rules and laws however being cruel and judgmental towards others who do so, irritable, disregarding safety of themselves or others, placing blame on others for what they do or how they treat them, lacking empathy.

Biological men have a higher diagnosis of NPD and a history of adverse childhood experiences. However, borderline person-ality disorders have a higher manifestation in biological women. There is a genetic and environmental aspect of this development. BPD can occur in biological males and because narcissistic person-ality is in the same cluster of disorders, there is a shared com-monality of behaviors, such as the fear of abandonment (real and imagined), impulsiveness, instability in relationships, anxiety, de-pression, dissociative aspects, dramatic shifts in perceptions of people and situations around them, and self harm or harm to others. They engage in bullying others and intimidating others and do not feel *genuine* remorse for what they do; however, they are very adept at acting and feigning remorse when it is in THEIR best interest to perform. They will blame others for what they do and may display patterns of excessive emotionality and atten-tion seeking. They then project their 'drama queen' behaviors onto others to control and manipulate them and are uncomfortable in situations where the attention is not on them. (This is when they may drink more, smoke more, sulk more).

They can be both vague and shallow, lacking detail and flir-tatious and seductive. They will say and do things to shame or embarrass you in casual meeting groups to one up you and dis-play what they perceive to be their power to control you. Their sense of entitlement is profound and they deem they should have special treatment. This is where their sense of self-worth and value derive. It is not intrinsic value but extrinsic and depends on external rewards. Their world comes crashing down when they are faced with the perception that they have human weaknesses and limitations. Admiration from others is so important they feel intense anger and shame and take it out on others. Their needs to be powerful and admired conflict with relationships where they are devoid of feeling real intimacy...even when they manipulate you to think otherwise. Their status and image comes before everything else because this is how they feel important. This is why they will shift from over idealizing you and others to devaluing you and others. They alter between feelings of deflation and worthlessness to bolstering their bravado and expect admiration from others to support their fragile self esteem. This is why they can be manipulative.

Although they *can* hide their true face from others for a *time*, they *will* make sure that if we have a safe place outside of their control...they will control it. They will strive to also control the access to other persons who you consider emotionally supportive and safe in some way. Their power over you demands that you are leverage to other people who want to encourage you to stand up against their abuse.

During childhood, if the narcissist is a parent, you are just one of those *troubled* kids that rescuers reach out to 'help' because something is 'clearly wrong with you' as they will say. Although people can exhibit these traits at times, for them these traits are inflexible and regularly observed, and cause functional impairment in intra/interpersonal relationships, work, school, home. An estimated 90% of mothers are either abused, or witness abuse, and according to the Child First Campaign, '40-70 percent of children' are *direct* victims of abuse in the home. As an adult or young woman, your brain has been hijacked by a tool called *love bombing* (keep reading I will get to that one too). (Smaller children also experience lovebombing more until they reach the age where they do not idolize the parent at all costs, and are trying to naturally seek independence from the parent).

A narcissistic abuser makes sure to trap you before he/she really shows their spots. Isolation is part of *their* conditioning. (Think about how many times you have been moved, Dear Alice, away from family who protected you or told your family or friends, who you hung out with were the issue when they were healthy influences or your safe places).

One allegation is that you provoke their response. No, Dear Alice's, you do not 'provoke' the narcissistic abuser. You are not to blame for the choices of someone to choose to abuse or demean you. Blaming you for their responsibility is unhealthy toxic abuse.

Narcissistic abuse is psychological *and* emotional. Narcissistic abusers are masters at using coercive control, psychological and physical abuse, emotional and sexual abuse, harassment, stalking, and online digital abuse.

The role of *headship* does not involve domineering abuse or manipulative coercion. It does not allow harsh conditioning abuse and unwarranted angry punishment because children act in ways a father or mother do not approve. It is vehement evil seeking to kill, steal from you, or destroy you, and are often dressed as mentors or pillars in the community, community leaders, deacons, ministers, Bishops, Elders, fathers, mothers, stepparents, lovers, teachers, stars you look up to. Narcissistic abusers are dressed in various elegant clothes and even seem presentable, all together, *seem* safe, secure, charming. We can look to Ted Bundy, Anders Breivik, pastor what's his face, and even persons called 'dad' or 'mom' who all share the same underlying sociopathy or narcissistic abuse. Narcissistic abuse is *all about* power and control. THEY are not able to have self awareness, reflection, or genuine empathy for others.

Each encounter with you creates a different file folder of a memory, a different rabbit hole or path in Wonderland...a different table of tea time. You try to plan how to manage the pain. Each way looks odd, and you may feel like escape is hopeless. It is nonsense to want to *feel* safe and secure. When you remember to be brave, you stick up for yourself...until you are undermined by the continuous reinforcement of shame. If you manage to cry, or when because of 'too much too much too much' negative energy inside of the traumatized memory neural network, you are halted and ridiculed about your display. The narcissistic abuser, the pawns in the narcissist's game, those who have not healed from narcissistic abuse themselves (and are reflecting it), and your inner negative cognitions all are screaming at you to *stop crying like this*! You are left feeling *isolated, alone, desperate. You 'almost think' you 'remember feeling a little different.'* However, you *'are not the same.'* So, who in the world ARE you?

Seeking proper assistance in healing from traumatic events (*not merely talking to a friend or family member who may be very limited in knowledge of scope and practice of healing from clinical levels of complex narcissistic abuse and trauma*) is vital. Often much is withheld in family/friend/girlfriend group 'therapy' because fear has been maladaptively (*negatively*) encoded into a self-dialogue the narcissist has made sure to drive home: that 'no one will believe' you, you 'deserved the treatment,' or 'must have done something to contribute to...' whatever was done abusively towards you. (*This is gaslighting and an abusive tactic*).

The residual effects of emotional and psychological abuse are serious. These types of abuses escalate to physical abuse and violence. Domestic violence survivors keep secrets of their abuser. Loyalty is a trait they rely on. The tools used during psychological and emotional relationships have occurred in such a way the survivor connects with negative self-cognitions that yell and scream inner thoughts 'this is not so bad,' 'I was overreacting,' and 'at least he/she didn't hit me.' (Until they do, and then when they do hit you, it will be *'your fault'* according to their narrative). It is not about 'spanking' in childhood...it is about *abuse.* Parents who spank are *not* necessarily abusive or narcissistic abusers. Although it is more frowned upon culturally and socially currently, spanking is smacking a child on one's buttocks with an open hand, and not with excessive force, and is to be reasonable and moderate as discipline, not leaving bruises, scratches, cuts with open hands, or with weapons (as according to the law). Once a blow leaves a mark on a child's body, it is considered legally in various states and countries, abuse. Abuse involves willful and intentional harm that leads to physical, mental, emotional, and sexual injuries.

The difference is the method of *discipline* from a calm mind, that is teachable, calm, and dignified. Punishment is not harsh or punitive abuse. Abuse is the opposite of all of calmness, or dignity. Therefore, when I speak of narcissistic abusers, I speak of violators who physically abuse, emotionally abuse, manipulate, ignore boundaries, are dismissive of you and your feelings, and critical in speech, actions, and behaviors (parents and or those you are romantically involved with). Abuse occurs in childhood and adulthood with persons who are narcissistic partners or parents. They can hide behind the cloak of social status, and position. Not all are privileged. What is the same is the feeling of being left drowning in an ocean of your own tears (and fears).

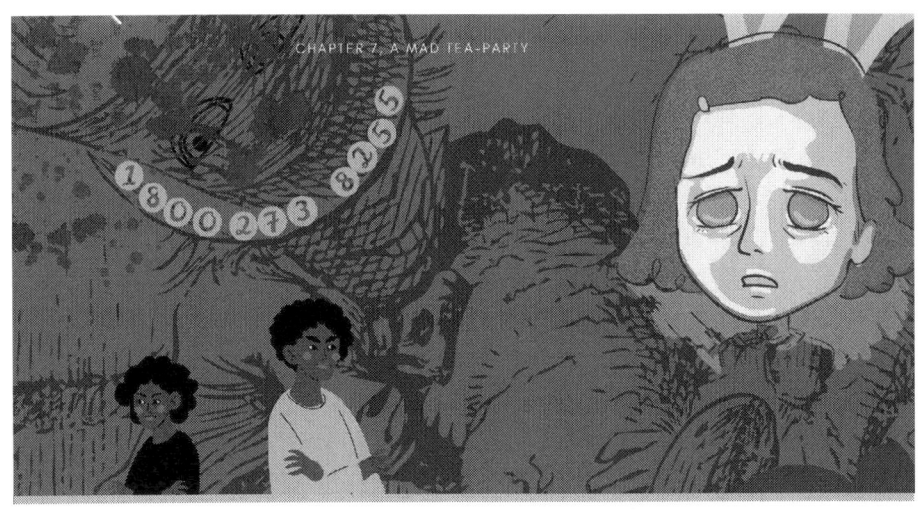

CHAPTER THREE

A Long Tail to Find the Way

In my culture, women are precious creations placed here by God (Psalms 139, NASB), and chosen by Him for *His* purpose (Jer. 29:11, NASB). A Biblical Truth for those of you reading this who identify as Christian: Jesus *protected* women! He did not scorn, demean, ridicule, dominate, manipulate, or abuse in *any* of His examples for men to women OR to parents over children! Oppositional to His example is a narcissistically abusive relationship (childhood or adulthood), where you feel isolated and want to just disappear right away. Many forms of childhood trauma occur in *isolated* environments infrequently witnessed by others affecting women (and men) to the core of their *relational* being.

A relationship is a connection amid two or more persons. It can be romantic, platonic, familial, or any other type of bond. In the United States, one in four women experiences, or has already experienced, violence within one or more of these types of relationships. According to WHO, worldwide, '1 in 3 (30%) of women' *have been* subjected to physical and/or sexual intimate partner violence or non-partner sexual violence within their lifetime. Also among this statistic is one third (27%) of women aged 15-49 years having been in a violent relationship with one of the above examples of relationships. According to the United Nations, violence against women is globally defined as '*any act of gender-based violence*' resulting in, '*or is likely to result in, physical, sexual, or mental harm or suffering to women,*' and this further includes threats of acts, coercion, arbitrary deprivation of liberty, whether occurring in public or within one's private life (WHO, 2022).

As children, we are self aware of events, afraid, and burdened by a sense of stigmatization, humiliation, culpability, or self-blame. Individuals undergoing traumatic events such as childhood physical, psychological, or sexual abuse may not understand that what has happened to them. The label abuse is erroneous and many women cannot label events as 'abuse' or experiencing 'victimization' (Maxfield, 2014). WHO notes when children grow up in families where there is violence, they suffer a range of behavioral and emotional disturbances associated with perpetrating or experiencing violence later throughout one's lifetime. Childhood traumas that are intra (*deep relational* oriented), interpersonal (*surface level* oriented), intentional, and chronic are associated with greater rates of severe anxiety disorders, antisocial behaviors, and increased risk for alcohol and substance use disorders (Maxfield, 2014). When we undergo traumas during childhood, we experience massive alterations in brain development, due to the brain's high levels of plasticity during childhood and it can carry over into adulthood when not addressed in trauma recovery therapy. Sometimes you feel you will '*never get to twenty at this rate.*' (Carroll, L, 1865).

During exposure to chronic stressors, the brain mandates

a diverse production of responses. Some responses mobilize energy production, while other responses increase cardiovascular activity or decrease unnecessary physiological processes (Maxfield, 2014). Words do not come the same as they used to, and during childhood, may not have been encoded to begin with in that memory! Some memories happened before you were able to talk or have rational cognition of your feelings or ability to say no. Long term trauma of narcissistic abuse disturbs the development of the brain, decreasing the hippocampal dimensions which "may be related to the fragmentation of memory that occurs…and…dissociation" (Maxfield, 2014, p. 1). This affects the brain by producing deficits and damage within emotional, behavioral, cognitive, and social functioning (Maxfield 2014). You feel alone and tired and frightened about your own changes.

Complex Trauma

Long-lasting exposures to traumatic stress affect how we, as children manage our environment on a systematic foundation affecting biological, psychological, sociological, and spiritual response (De Bellis, Spratt, & Hooper, 2011). The limbic system, for example, monitors emotion, memory, and behavior within the central nervous system. This system is indispensable for self-preservation. Trauma causes limbic abnormalities in the amygdala and hippocampus by hijacking inclusive flight or fight responses the body uses to regulate stress inducing triggers. The amygdala is what is responsible in the brain for preparing the body for action.

During an event that is traumatic to a child, the amygdala responds *too quickly* for the cerebral cortex to consider potential trigger mechanisms as threats. This prevents the **body** from being able to *choose* which fight or flight response is appropriate against the antagonist. Because of excess and adverse neurobiological results of events occur within the trauma, de-activation of a child's prefrontal cortex occurs. This is imperative within a bio-psycho-social-spiritual aspect and within healing from early or adolescent childhood abuse by a parent with narcissistic domineering traits because the prefrontal cortex is responsible for the brain's executive functioning. Executive functioning regulates planning, problem solving, organizing, and directing the child's body to perform daily activities. The door shuts on us being able to 'talk' about it when language is compromised in the encoded traumatic events.

Complex trauma events differ broadly and comprise of physical, sexual, emotional abuses, neglect, observing domestic violence, and exposures to external environmental violence, and medical trauma. You fall into the perpetually endless abyss of the sea of tears, feel punished, and suppose that you will drown in your own tears. Impairment associated with complex trauma exposure range from inadequacies in relationships, attachment disorders, emotional and behavioral dysregulations and development of personality disorders such as borderline and histrionic, cognitive/attentional failures, and biological fluctuations that affect children's overall physical health, including vitamin deficiencies.

As adolescents we experience dissociation, undergo variations of our own self-perception. We identify alterations in our individual worldview...but hurt people hurt people. In states of dysregulation which are foundational in narcissistic abuse, we can drive people away from us who genuinely care. (This is often the *plan* of the narcissistic abuser because they *want you* to feel alone to depend on them so they can have supply).

Like Alice who encountered a mouse while swimming in the pool of her own tears in Lewis Carroll's (1865) versions, we continue to offend those trying to connect with us. When others relate to us their tales, their fears, there can be a tendency to take on 'too much too much' from them in return because the narcissistic abuser is covertly conditioning us to rescue *them* from their consequences and avoid accountability to justify their abuse. The result of their conditioning is for us to feel *responsible* for their temper tantrums and rage. We feel like the mouse with a long tale, condemned to death by the Judge and Jury, the Cunning Fury.

Complex trauma occurs during developmental caregiving relationships that initially form our principles about self and the world, such as is the world safe, or unsafe? Do I have the ability to feel secure? However, abuse involves development of negative self-perceptions that become distorted acknowledgements, such as a perception "I am...worthless." These negative self-perceptions become 'factual' statements of self and are called *maladaptive* (because they are negative self-statements) that have power to encode negative perceptions of self and replay over and over in future reminders of the originally encoded memory event.

We cultivate *maladaptive* distorted ascriptions to try and cope with the abusive trauma, our environment, and resulting indicators, such as believing we deserve to be abused. According to Kliethermes, Schacht, and Drewry "...Maladaptive beliefs may build a foundation for impaired social interactions and further mental health deficits" (Kliethermes, Schacht, and Drewry, 2014, p. 345). The biological effects of trauma reduce our awareness of our bodies, manifesting as somatic symptoms, amplifying electrical irritability within our limbic structures, and lead to severe "...Long-term health risk behaviors and diseases" (Kliethermes, Schacht, and Drewry, 2014, p. 346).

Physical abuse is in no way an easy thing to deal with. Emotional and psychologically abusive traumas are just as powerful in the brain and body connection as a physical blow because negative (maladaptive) memories encode a deeper response to self-negative cognitions. When asked what I do, I once responded to a parent "I listen to others and encourage them (in love) to delve into the recesses of their inner mirrors like *Atreyu* from "*The Neverending Story*," and together, we face the destruction of the mind's inner '*Nothing's*' as destructive forces while leading them out of the inner rabbit holes from mad places of their mind, like Alice, stuck within a madhouse of a nightmare." *(Yes that book IS coming soon)*. This includes the madness of having survived abusive relationship(s). I intentionally used plural form for relationships because with abuse, there is not just one abusive relationship...what is discovered is a long stemming pattern of abuse stemming from early childhood or adolescence into young adulthood.

For many women, the pain is not on display to the outside world from psychological abuse...put your head up high and pretend you don't see the demons roaming in this sky! We are perceived through temperament or stereotyping of roles as *'strong.'* The word *'strong'* has so many various cultural pressures attached, and is not limited to one culture or demographic over others. As 'survivors' part of the survival adaptation to shield 'self' from an unsafe world involves the need to hide those inner most scars because of intense feelings of isolation and control from the person who is abusive. Therefore, we cannot afford to let others see what is really going on *in secret.* What they *will see* will be the ways we try to cope with the trauma through substance abuse, self harm, suicidal ideation, shopping and hoarding behaviors for some, gambling, for some, sex. Whatever way we feel we can have a sense of control (even when it is dysfunctional and irrational) is what we will do. Whatever is our response to trauma, we will use. Recall that trauma changes and prevents our ability to use rational thought of behavior. We become emotionally dysregulated. If we are fight response prone we will fight. If we are flight response prone, we will run, hide, flee to get away. If we are freeze response prone, we will become unable to speak or immobile when we are attacked and anxiety prone to provocation. Then there is the fawn effect where we stay in a loop of I 'should or could have done' something. The irrational behaviors are behaviors that seek *pleasure* (that is what we were originally created to pursue) however, now we have a negative consequence: Addictions. We need to feel good...and so we do whatever we can in our desperation to feel something...our brain has been hijacked AND it does not have the ability to regulate what we *should* do that is healthy. In childhood, we do what we think we should do...because as children we do not know rationally what an outcome is from an adult mindset.

The brain eventually *leaks* regardless of how *'strong'* we think we are. We can only store so much negative energy in our mind...(negative thoughts are neurons and are energy, and are stored). We can only *pretend* to be *'mad'* (which is normal in Won-

derland), for so long before we feel we are too, or SHOULD be, and so we need to forget our own muchness and uniqueness. We need to learn to be like everyone else in wonderland, no matter how twisted they are. Our brain *encodes* these events and we do not chose where it stores it.

Adaptive events do not bother us or negatively leak or cause irrational thoughts or behaviors. *Maladaptive* events do. Consider your brain. Nerve impulses are responsible for moving along a neuron then to neighborhoods (twisted paths) along other neurons (throughout wonderland). A signal from one upstream of one neuron to another encourages another neighbor downstream to send a code on to another neighbor or to stop it from continuing down *that* path while some neurons go faster than others...because it is an electrical impulse.

Trauma events are maladaptive events and so trauma events not only rewire the brain, **but it also overloads it**. This is when, in my office, I see patients who are presenting with various levels of anxiety and depression...which are fear based and tied to maladaptively (negative) encoded events in the neural network, and addictions. They are stuck in unhealthy relationships and not able to leave. Their muchness is lost. Their minds are trapped in Twisted Wonderland. *Which way, which way, which way* the brain screams when it is overloaded and short circuited by *too much too much too much sadness*!

When we are presented a situation that reminds our brain's encoded files of a former event driving our minds we can quickly go through those early encoded responses between our brain and body and feel out of control on the inside, mentally screaming all over our body that *it's teatime all the time, Alice! You're mad! OFF with your head you stupid girl!* Even in situations that are safe, our brain's (*rational*) mind-body connection sends irrational responses that tell our body to respond instead of a rational positive thought with the screaming mad voices *"I am NOT safe!", "I'm not good enough!", "I should have known better!", "I cannot trust anyone!", "I am powerless/helpless!"*
These negative cognitions (and there are plenty more) drive us

through a Twisted Wonderland of madness…and over and over you feel like you are meeting people who want to chop off your head, threaten your life, or want you trapped at the same tea party over and over with no resolve. You find yourself abandoned by Time to be at the tea table with the March Hare and the Dormouse, because the narcissistic abuser wants to control you, then throw you away to keep your mind guessing how to please him/her at the cost of your mind, at the cost of your muchness, Dear Alice, and at the cost of your mental stability. You are *mad!*

Like Alice, you may feel as though you have fallen down a hole, chasing an interesting rabbit who caught your eye of curiosity one day *because the person looked safe*, was *supposed to be* safe because of a family relationship, looked or seemed interesting, or drew your attention by intentionally placing him or herself in your direct line of sight to target you. You feel one way, and then the other. You wonder, like Alice, *how did I get this way? How did I fall? What's happening to me? 'You and your abuse you're so much worse than anything she could ever say! To be so big that I kick you away! Sometimes she ran because it was not safe to stay. But where did she go but down an endless way?'* (My Heart My Broken Heart, Buchanan, 2022).

You feel as though your world is…*mad.*

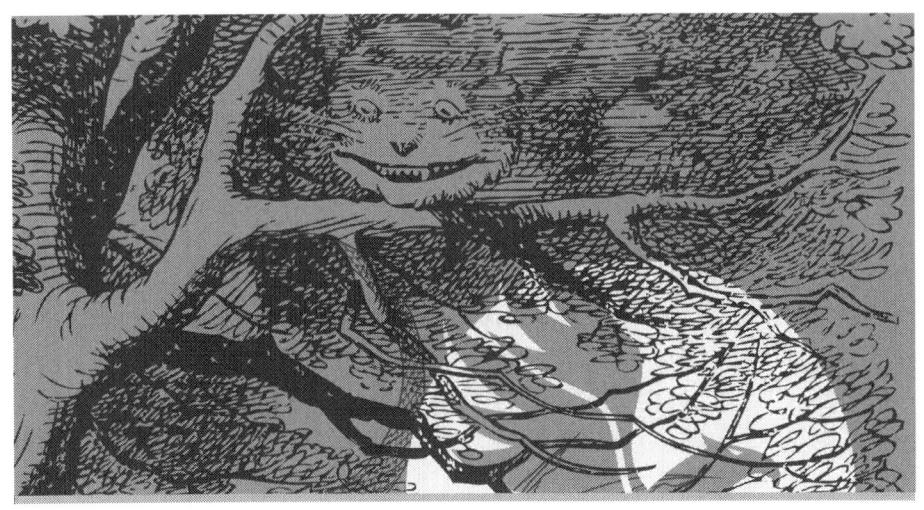

CHAPTER FOUR

Cheshire Cat

"A Cheshire cat appears...like mist of a fog. She's silent but deadly sitting on the tree a few yards off. The cat only grins and smiles at my back. She disappears when I ask her the way out. She casts me aside and sends me back out. To get attacked by the Jabberwocky who lurks all about" (Buchanan, 2022).

The Cheshire Cat serve two roles in Twisted Wonderland. He/She is a twisted pawn, and an *elemental* aspect of trauma. As a pawn of a narcissistic dominant parent, for example, one parent/ or you as the romantic partner act as an intermittent reinforcer. The narcissist has trauma bonded in his or her relationship and one weapon that is healthy is positive (*reinforcing*) behaviors from the narcissist (*from time to time*). However, this tool called the Cheshire Cat is unhealthy because this is leaving you in a continuous cycle of trying to de-code what it is *they* want to keep getting from you.

What they want is obedience and complete submission without question *at all costs*. They want for you to bend your value systems to please them...at all costs. For children, this means trying to figure out which parent to approach for common requests. For romantic partners, this means one thing they want from you is to have dominance in the bedroom, or in public when around the persons they chose for you to be around. They need for you to obey them at all costs...and the Cheshire Cat is a mental yo-yo. One minute you are okay and the next minute you are wondering how to disappear to placate their anger.

Setbacks or negative behaviors follow periods where the waves of adoring treatment come. This keeps you hooked on trying to figure out how to please the abuser(s) and get back into their good graces once again.

The narcissistic parent(s)/lovers are emotionally abusive because of their *impossible* constantly evolving demands and expectations. They lack self-awareness and empathy for others, including children and are highly sensitive and defensively explosive. This takes a toll on your mental health. They may brag about what you achieve as it makes them also look good publicly; however, emotional support is not provided and the flip flop from publicly well liked to harsh critical, controlling and over demandingness keeps you spinning.

They will use their spouse (if they are a parent) or use a disappearing act to negatively motivate you by assuming 'good cop bad cop' scenario or I want you no I don't want you scenario, as the Cheshire Cat incarnate. The narcissistic parent(s)or romantic partner will misinterpret assertiveness and healthiness as an *attack* against them. Then they will project their own feelings of '*I am unworthy*' onto (children or)/you along with *their own* internalized negative traits of attention seeking and selfishness and ignore the needs of (children's)/your feelings and emotions through claims of YOU being emotionally weak, overdramatizing your emotions, or too sensitive to their 'jokes' and emotional strings and detached perspectives of genuine emotional intimacy.

The insecurity projected onto children/you by forcing them/you to stifle feelings and needs to abate the narcissistic parent/lover creates insecurity and teaches them/you the message to learn is "*love is* **conditional.**" (SIDEBAR: NOW for you readers who are '*Christians,*' consider what THIS does to a child when they are told to consider God is *love!*) LOVE MEANS CONDITIONS to them/you because that is their/your conditioned reality and their/your normality. This negatively affects relationships with others. One of the (*many*) maladaptively encoded self-thoughts throughout childhood that leaks into adulthood is "*I'm not good enough*" due to the internalized belief *you* are the issue, are selfish, and responsible for how the narcissistic responds or 'just is.' *Love is conditional* is your message.

The *non-narcissistic parent* has the potential to absorb the dominant narcissistic parents' traits. The parent who is *codependent* is unable to separate themselves and their own self-identity from the dominant narcissistic parent. **Lack of protection can be more traumatic than the trauma of the abuse**, and rarely will the narcissistic parent engage cooperatively in teamwork (for long) due to the constant need for admiration and to *be* and feel powerful. There is a strong tie to codependency in parental relationships.

It may seem like an unintentional backhanded comment about food...the dishes, the color you picked for the wall, how you decorated the living room, failed to pay attention, how you wrecked the car 'on purpose' because you are a terrible driver, failed to put gas in the car because you are incompetent, or the car needs maintenance. You, parents, also become a tool of a narcissistic parent...you become the *Cheshire Cat.* You try to explain it was not your intention to be forgetful, or to not pick a neutral color, or forgot to stop and get gas. However, the narcissistic abuser *Time* is off on a tangent of RAGE.

In this rage, you are being programmed too…to feel unhinged and berated. You feel scolded and want to disappear yourself, to go back into the background and push the narcissist onto someone else…absent mindedly. The narcissist will throw things in your face too, *Cheshire Cat*. They will target you and berate you for their perception of you coming against them should you choose to defend Twisted Alice or help Twisted Alice traverse out of Twisted Wonderland. You learn to do so covertly…you learn to be a covert narcissist. Their stare will frighten you…it is full of rage and when they posture, all you want to do even when you are a fighter is fade away. They use the silent treatment to punish you, Cat. They will demand an apology to fake their way out. Time has a history of cutting you out…it may start with the gas and end with the bills. It seems like a gift, but Time must have control because to them it thrills. They will dump their issues onto you too. They will accuse you of lying whenever they are through. They are trapped in their own Twistedness and will blame you Cheshire's for trying to help others get out. Time is the victim…in this you must know that he/she is always right, and Cheshire Cat, you must obey like so.

Cheshire Cat Of Codependent Parents

Narcissistic parents/person will put their emotional needs ahead of their children/you *and* will expect for you/or their spouse to be on their side at all costs to sustain provisions afforded in the relationship against others including children. In addition to the narcissistic parent emotionally abandoning their children, there is an expectation to listen to their rants and rages, and for their children to follow suit or else. It is a *conditioned response to trauma* that says, 'oh that is just the way so and so is…you know to just ignore it.' They judge and expect excellence and place unrealistic expectations for "you *should do…instead*' and this further alienates members of the family unit. Codependence is enmeshment. They fail to see for themselves HOW the decisions mandated by the narcissistic parent ensures the child(ren), and

even the adult child's decisions because control and over depend-
ance is what the narcissistic parent wants at all costs because that
is power for them.

The codependent parent also serves in this way a *Cheshire Cat*
role, not really telling the child which way is safe, all the while vic-
ariously serving the narcissistic parent by slyly relaying "I don't
know which way is the way out...or how (the child) can find *their*
way' (any other way opposite of the control of Time in other
words). "She does not know how I can find my way. It depends
a good deal, she says on which way (you) want to define (your)
way..." with a sly grin. The codependent parent will often toss you
aside and send you back out...to get attacked by the Jabberwocky
(narcissist's temper) who lurks all about. *'They're both mad, she
says with a sneer. We're all mad here girl, why didn't you KNOW
that by then!'* This is because there is an encoded engrained programmed fear in leaving the narcissist and the abusive relationships. They require someone who caters to their needs and who
will give up their own desires (even to help their children). It is to
be peace at all costs, Cheshire Cat...and this manipulated purpose
is because *Time* controls *you* too...and at the cost of children of
narcissists.

Time may not abuse the Cheshire Cat directly in all cases...
but Time does require supply *and a servant.* The Cheshire Cat role
serves the narcissist in that the Cheshire Cat must be a subject
and a cohort. Time will not accept the Cheshire Cat being different either. Time violates the Cheshire Cat's boundaries, tracks the
Cheshire Cat's locations, becomes over involved in the Cheshire
Cat's work and hobbies. Time controls the Cheshire Cat's dress, demeanor, place, and image in the public eye.

Time also plays the role of the victim *and* influences the
Cheshire Cat to riddle others in pain, to gain sympathy and attention using the Cheshire Cat as supply. The Cheshire Cat is
not always immune to the cruelness of Time's idealizations devalu-
ations, and love bombing. Narcissist's are well versed in praise
and attention to keep the Cheshire Cat from disappearing on
them. (Time has abandonment issues stemming from childhood

that do not go away). The subtle games they play at learning to control confuses others and leaves you, Dear Alices, and you, Cheshire Cat's, jumping through hoops (or trees) over and over. They will *'spin spin spin'* to alter your own perception, Cheshire Cat, of 'who' in Twisted Wonderland is also trapped and a bit... mad!

"OH, YOU CAN'T HELP THAT,' SAID THE CAT. 'WE'RE ALL MAD HERE."
The Toll of the Cheshire Cat as Depersonalization and Derealization in Trauma

The treatment of psychological trauma varies with emotional issues presented, and how the brain has encoded memories into the mind and body connection. Providing cognitive and behavioral treatment in therapy (*not a friend group*) assists the brain and body to connect to identify emotional meanings of trauma, and how various maladaptive events (traumas) are linked to fear, anxiety, and depression (Franklin, 2011). The brain body connection has three defense mechanisms that are created to help us handles stressors. These responses are defense mechanisms that activate diverse neurochemicals, triggers and reminders of the memories with a connection to what the brain tells the body to do as far as movement during an attack. Not all attacks will encode the same response, and often there is a mixture of the three responses together.

The fight-flight-freeze responses are defense mechanisms each person's brain and body use to protect from *'perceived'* danger. SOMETIMES the brain gets overloaded and non-threatening situations can be perceived (by the brain body connection) as threatening. When your brain grabs on to a memory of the same threatened feeling, fight-flight-freeze responses are automatically (by themselves) triggered, and many bodily-physiological changes prepare you to confront (*fight*), run away (*flight*), or freeze you in place when there is a person, situation, or environment the brain perceives as a threat.

The **Fight** response activates: Tightened jaws, tight fists, clenched teeth, desire to strike someone or something, wanting to kick or punch, glaring, raised voice, feeling of nausea, knots in stomach, homicidal or suicidal thoughts, anger, rage, crying, hands in fists, grinding teeth, snarling, fight in eyes and voice, desires to stomp and kick, burning stomach, use of metaphors like bombs and volcanoes.

The **Flight** response activates: Anxiousness, shallow breathing, rapid moving darting eyes, not able to focus, restless movements in limbs, fidgeting, feeling trapped, feeling tense, feeling restless legs, numb in legs, big darting eyes, leg and foot movements, fidgety-ness, feeling trapped, tense, sense of running in life and excessive exercise.

The **Freeze** response activates: Feeling stuck in the body, cold/numb, paling skin, sweating, stiffness, heaviness in the limbs, decreased heart rate, increase in heart rate, orientation to threats, restricted breathing and holding of the breath, sense of dread and foreboding, fawning, people pleasing behaviors, conflict avoidance, unable to find your voice to be assertive over aggressiveness, taking care of the needs of others over self needs to a point of unhealthy toxic behaviors.

These defense mechanisms are triggered when threats occur as according to memories that have been previously programmed in our storage and are retrieved to reactivate at times the brain and body are reminded of similar triggers and situations to emotional well-being. An *'Event'* is the encoded memory of fear having been programmed in memory storage, for example, embarrassment or shame before giving a presentation and the body experiencing 'stage fright' as a triggered *Fight-Flight-Freese* response. In events during each person's lifetime, symptoms may do more harm than good when responding to present and future events. An increased heart rate and sweating might help someone escape from a bear; however, it does not help the same person experience overcoming perceived fear of danger during a public presentation or speaking up assertively when called vulgar or hateful names when someone does not get their way and bullies you through narcissistic gaslighting or saying assertively 'do not hit me or touch me' during a physical altercation or batterer situation with a narcissistic abuser.

Everyone experiences fight-flight-freeze responses at various life events when the brain encodes memories to varying degrees. It can be natural, healthy, and some events that bother others may not bother all persons the same way...just as Alice's reactions to seeing a white rabbit in clothes did not cause her to be shocked; whereas, it may have caused another person to feel shocked. However, when fight-flight-freeze responses leads to excessive anger, prolonged stress, anxiety, depression, trauma, and other co-occurring medical problems, (such as excess stress, high blood pressure, unhealthy eating, unhealthy lifestyle choices in handling emotions and memories), it is called maladaptive and stores negative thoughts (that are also neurons, neurons being a form of energy). *'A Cheshire cat appears ...like mist of a fog. She's silent but deadly sitting on the tree a few yards off.'* (Buchanan, 2022). Symptoms of (post-traumatic stress disorder) PTSD from narcissistic abuse, embody behavioral manifestations of stress-induced changes in brain structure and function.

Narcissists help others and even provide them favors as favors provide them with power over those they help...you owe them something. *'She does not know how I can find my way. It depends a good deal she says, on which way I want to define my way.'* (Buchanan, 2022). Nothing is given without an attachment or condition. They will abuse this power dynamic without remorse and string you along by using it as leverage and demanding more than the initial favor was even worth. The price comes with interest, and they will continually remind you how much 'they' helped and 'did this' for you 'when you (blank)' (using a backhanded compliment and insult to degrade you). They will guilt you to seek a position of power and hurting you does not preclude their abuse as they do not experience empathy for you as a person of equal rank.

Narcissistic abusers are motivated by feeling superior over others, and adulation, fame, influence, opportunities, notoriety, and additional resources only entrench your mind in confusion. They will act *'kind'* to you after you are discarded only because they want something from you. Survivors of narcissistic abuse struggle to overcome traumatic reactions months and years of being denigrated and told how much 'trouble' 'stupid' 'useless' 'worthless' they are. After years of gaslighting and manipulation, this increases feelings of anxiety and depression. You struggle because you do not know what the abuser is going to do next. Your brain remains on constant alert in chronic hypervigilance and expecting them to be around every corner. You struggle with feeling safe and secure, because situations, places, and people remind you of the abuse. *'They're both mad, she says with a sneer. We're all mad here, girl, why didn't you know that by then!'*

The brain encodes bodily responses for past, present, future references. Our future events during each event may are encoded the same way and our brain's neural network places *each* memory as a file folder compartmentalizing rabbit holes of events for later retrieval. When a memory event is *adaptively* encoded, we feel safe no matter the event. We feel positive about interactions with persons in the event. We feel positive about the location of the event. We feel positive about bodily responses and sensory responses in the event. For example, one child is abused yet, the other child is not present, does not hear the abuse, is themselves are not abused. One child faces a *jabberwocky* in a nightmare Wonderland of Twistedness while the other child experiences Wonderland as the greatest place ever. This is why siblings have alternate perceptions of childhoods when abuse has taken place and when they have narcissistic parent(s). The Cheshire Cat did not appear to both children...only to one.

The brain areas associated with our stress response comprises of our amygdala, hippocampus, and prefrontal cortex (Butcher, Hooley, Mineka, 2014). Traumatic stress is associated with long-term variations in these areas, chronic exposure to continuous onslaught, and programming with intervals of 'honeymoon' periods because narcissistic abusers need to *appear* helping, caring, and can get others to cheer them on for being a *'nice'* person. *'The cat only grins and smiles at my back. She disappears when I ask her the way out. She casts me aside and sends me back out.'*

When the brain encodes an event maladaptively, the brain retrieves memories, bodily responses, self-thoughts, energy, environment, and people as symbology of who we are around or involved with at the time of the event. It responds according to our unique temperament blend, attachment style at random times when triggered by internal or external reminders to ANY encoded threat in the memory file. This is when underlying issues re-occur, and eventually grow worse and unhealthy as far as coping behaviors. The emotional and bodily response leaks out in some way... and we experience further unhealthy coping mechanisms, traumatic stress, and avoidance to attempt to alleviate what we feel.

Thoughts are neurons. Thoughts are energy. Energy gets stored within our inner most rooms of our mind in files that harbor people, environmental triggers, emotional and bodily responses, self-thoughts that drive either positive or negative replays, and reminders that keep grabbing us and sucking us down into the abyss of the same dark rabbit holes over and over...stuck in *Time's* everlasting loop.

Cheshire Cat Of Dissociation And Depersonalization

Our psyche even takes on a life of a *Cheshire Cat*...as we learn to automatically disassociate or disappear from normality, or reality of what is occurring to us. Both dissociation and depersonalization can occur in trauma. Dissociation begins with nerve cells firing in sync at the same time. It creates a sense of being outside of one's body and often looking in...Alice looking into the mirror of herself on the other side. It can be disruptive, troubling to cope with, and chronic (ongoing). You ask what is self? Who *am I* girl? This perception of being on the outside looking in and not able to control self.

Temporarily you detach from self because of the region of the cortex responsible for keeping you tethered to who you are, which way you are going (*in PTSD Dissociation, we are not speaking* of DID, *Dissociative Identity Disorder and I have heard many clients attempting to self-diagnose themselves as DID when they are experiencing dissociation in trauma. Please do not self-diagnose as the two are diverse psychopathologies that share commonalities of this presentation*).

Dissociation in trauma is the brain attempting to adapt itself as a defense mechanism to highly stressful provoking circumstances and characterized by memory lapse, because of the amygdala's effect on the hippocampus and prefrontal cortex, with a sense of disconnection from oneself and one's surroundings. It can occur in our emotions, body sensations, memories, senses and can occur in situations that are also non-threatening because of the over-activated flight/fight reactions and the response of the amygdala that can become addicted to the dopaminergic adrenal response due to the amygdala role in fear. *'A Cheshire cat appears ... like mist of a fog. She's silent but deadly sitting on the tree a few yards off.'*

The amygdala is in charge of storing the VISUAL images of trauma as sensory fragments...and the memory here is not stored like a story, but rather, HOW the five senses experienced the various events *at the Time*
each one occurred. They are stored fragmentally through visual images, smells, sounds, tastes, what we experienced as far as touch! When traumatic events over activate the amygdala FEAR responses become more intense. Therefore, we experience flashbacks and waking nightmares! Hypervigilance occurs with exaggerated startle responses, because the amygdala overreacts and norepinephrine is released but not adequality controlled by the prefrontal cortex, because, as *I* explain to clients in therapy, 'Miss Amy G. Dala' (*HINT at another of my own children's book's coming out for 2022*) has shut down the prefrontal cortex's ability to let her know she can be calm again.

As the root issue maladaptively intensifies, with increased narcissistic abuse, this is when it is mindfully healthy to seek psychotherapy to learn how to process these events in an adaptive way as it involves the most important person: ourselves, and what thoughts our brain locked onto and kept repeating in our daily lives. This is the forever tunnel of the rabbit hole we can become lost in...regardless of the choices and behaviors of others, we are the only ones who can stop this cycle. We are individually, the only ones who can *choose* to learn which way leads to the escape of Twisted Wonderland. What we feel and experience is the overwhelming sense of just needing to somehow get '*Out of here out of this madness is the only answer I know! I don't know which way I don't care anymore! So long as I go somewhere safe away from this madness!'*

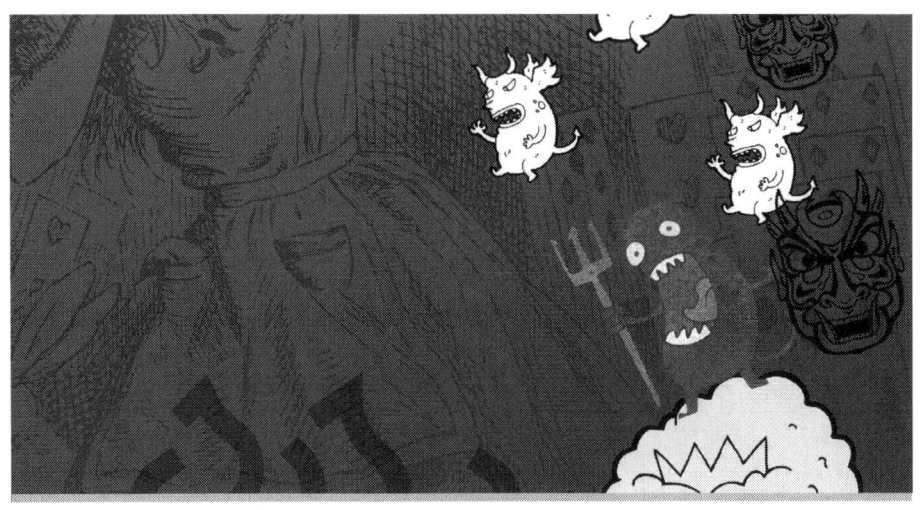

CHAPTER FIVE

The Rabbit Sends in Little Bill

A narcissistic parent/partner is a parent/partner influenced by narcissism or narcissistic personality disorder. Narcissistic parents/partner are solely and possessively close to their children/you and feel threatened by an adolescent's/your natural stage of growing independence and development. This results in a pattern of narcissistic attachment, wherein, the parent /partner believes the young person/you exists solely to fulfill his/her needs and desires. A narcissistic parent/partner will attempt to control through threats and emotional (often denigrating gaslighting) and emotional, psychological, and even physical abuse. Narcissistic parenting negatively affects the psychological development of adolescent's, affecting reasoning, emotional, ethical, and societal behaviors, and attitudes.

When experiencing narcissistic abuse, should a narcissist lose the mental hold or control they have over those in their circles they seek to dominate and have idolize them, they change tactics to gain control. They deny weaknesses. They overinflate their abilities. They will manipulate to control others while simultaneously belittling or criticizing you and then take credit for successes of positive actions the adolescent child or woman *may* accomplish. When their image publicly are *threatened* (in their perception) by *your* behaviors, they will let you have it. This is when you will see their rage. This is when their temper and violence escalate.

Like the white rabbit in Carroll's chapter 'The Rabbit Sends in Little Bill,' the rabbit will come looking for you. You will tremble in fear because their violence is unstable and the memories from their actions automatically trigger your amygdala to go into action within the fight/flight/freeze modalities. You will tremble and your mental house will be shaken. You will forget even when you grow larger that you are no longer small. That is what they rely on...putting you back into your place, *Dear Alice*, to control and manipulate you and drive you to forgetting your muchness so that only Twisted Alice is the one who responds in kind to their violence. They will come into the darkness of your inner most being right up the door of your sense of am I safe? Which way do I go to stay safe? They trap you in your waking nightmare. Physically, psychologically, and mentally, you are under attack.

When the narcissistic abuser(s) do not get a response, or you physically are hiding in a safe place, or blocking their way, they will go around and take a new tactic to find a back way. They will find an open window. When they cannot get at you either physically or psychologically, they will go out and find chess pawn recruits. These are recruits on their behalf consisting of others who have some sort of position, power, influence, and authority over you to draw you or *force* you out. This is why they use others you want to be close to against you. They will make sure they allow you on the surface to be close to them...unless those pawns defy them. They will seek to control them at all costs.

Like the White Rabbit, they will tell their underlings (even when the relationship seemingly is reciprocal between them), do this! NOW! She is not obeying! Break the glass! GET to her! Drag her out! MAKE him/her do what I say! They rely on the ones they control to do exactly what they want without question. DO NOT speak out against me. DO NOT defy my word is law. No one else's opinion matters, I am the only one who is right! You will all do what I say! They will continue to demand upon those they manipulate to get to you and when it does not work...they will entice them or manipulate them to burn down your mental house together!

When you remember to be brave, you may say 'If you do I will set Dinah on you!' You may scream and yell and act out once your fight mode has been activated...because the *Dinah* in your life is your safe place, the person *you* trust who will not be manipulated by them. They will make *sure* you are trapped (physically and psychologically) somewhere that Dinah is nowhere around. This is why they isolate you. Narcissistic abusers often have a pattern of moving areas, moving jobs. There is an engrained community excuse that it is for their job...and at the same time although it may be true, it allows the narcissistic abuser to avoid real intimacy and connection with others...although they will retain contact of those who supported them in those areas because they need supply. They need to know their supply will be there should they choose to relocate to that area in the future.

Narcissistic abusers have the ability to be very successful at what they do. They have the ability to be in positions of authority. They have the ability to find ways to increase their status. (Notice how these are not negative traits...what is negative is *how* these traits allow them to hide and how these traits are useful). They are drawn to areas they can be worshipped and looked up to. They need to feed their sense of *entitlement and* their public persona, and their private persona, are frighteningly different. They are able to put on a charade. One minute you see a nonthreatening white rabbit in a waistcoat with a pocket watch...the next the white rabbit changes into something far more demanding and re-jecting. They bounce from idealization to devaluation to rejection. This dynamic, *Dear Alice*, is meant to confuse you. This cycle of abuse is confounding and overwhelming.

First the narcissistic abuser will idealize you. This is the honeymoon stage where they manipulate you into their deep dark hole by thinking what a great person *they* are. They pour affection onto you. It feels great...at first. You have become emotionally attached. Then, the narcissistic abuser will shower you with little pebbles here and there...little jabs here and there while you are isolated to break you down.

You realize there may be red flags, and they are not stable, and they do not handle their mess in healthy ways. They are not so perfect. Their fur is not really White and clean...their clothes are not clean. They are really messy, dirty, and have very negative toxic habits. Very soon, the rabbit noticed Alice, and called out to her in an angry tone, 'Mary Ann!' go home now and serve me! Alice was so frightened she ran in the direction he said immediately he had pointed to without trying to even explain his mistake...she was not who he thought she was. (Not that it mattered because they are right at all costs). In his house she found a bottle labeled 'Drink Me.' She drank it just to see what the bottle did...anything to try and escape from Wonderland. She realized her safe place was much better than being lost in Wonderland. In a mournful tone she noted there was 'no room, no room to grow any more here.'

When the White Rabbit and his pawns of Little Bills throw pebbles at your face, they will hit you in your face. You can try and yell stop doing that and when you remember to be brave, for a mo-ment, it seems you have won. However, they are not shocked they are re-calculating their attacks against your defiance. If you can eat a cake like Alice does to find some way to grow small enough to escape maybe, you can find others who will help you. You may try and find a safe place to grow back to your normal size to feel okay again. However, they have ensured that although that is an excellent plan, neatly and simply arranged, the difficulty will be you not having the slightest idea how to set about it.

While you hide from their presence at least for a moment, anxiety has you peaking out among the trees, like little sharp bark over your head that causes you to look all about hypervigilant and hyperaroused at every noise and tremor you feel within the environment. Where can you go, *Dear Alice*, to feel safe in Twisted Wonderland? Narcissistic abusers do not let things go. They are seething and underlyingly consistently explosive when confronted with unmet expectations or perceived slight. They deny accountability for *their* actions and quickly turn the tables to blame others when confronted with assertive boundaries over the way they treat those who stand up to them. They are prone to easily exploding into fits of rage, overreacting, and becoming increasingly aggressive whenever they *feel* attacked by even the slightest criticism. The blame shifts to you as their victim when you or others on your side attempt to hold them accountable. Even though image wise, they project being a goodie-goodie and can be publicly charming or in their circles of those they have manipulated into overlooking their abusive qualities, they draw people to them in crowds. In their inner circles, conflict within the environment is experienced as external (and even covert aggressive).

Nothing is *their* fault. They hold on to unrealistic expectations they set onto others, and it is offensive to them when their unrealistic demands and authoritarian demeanors are not abiding by at any cost to you. They do not have the ability to feel genuine empathy. They fake it. They feign displaying genuine empathy at times; however, even their caregiving has a motivation. What they do must involve pleasing them at all costs.

Like the White Rabbit and Pat, they recruit others. The narcissist will recruit other servants, like Bill. Bill will be ordered to come and find you, Dear Alice, out of hiding. This is not because the White Rabbit cares about your feelings being hurt...it is because he needs another to do his/her bidding.

'When you dare to stand tall and not small that day, you will be sure to send Bill away, be wary, a mob will come hunting for you,

Dear Alice, that very day. Once the White Rabbit has located you, he will come for you with his demanding. You may hear broken glass and be snatched up unexpecting to to see from him such an angry danger-ous look. He has a temper too...a demanding voice that grows. His demeanor is distant and controlling and his temper grows. The first thing you will want to do is grow to your right size, you know. So you can escape the attack of the rocks hitting you in your face. You may find that in your running away, you come across a new face...that of the caterpillar sitting and waiting for you' (Buchanan, 2022).

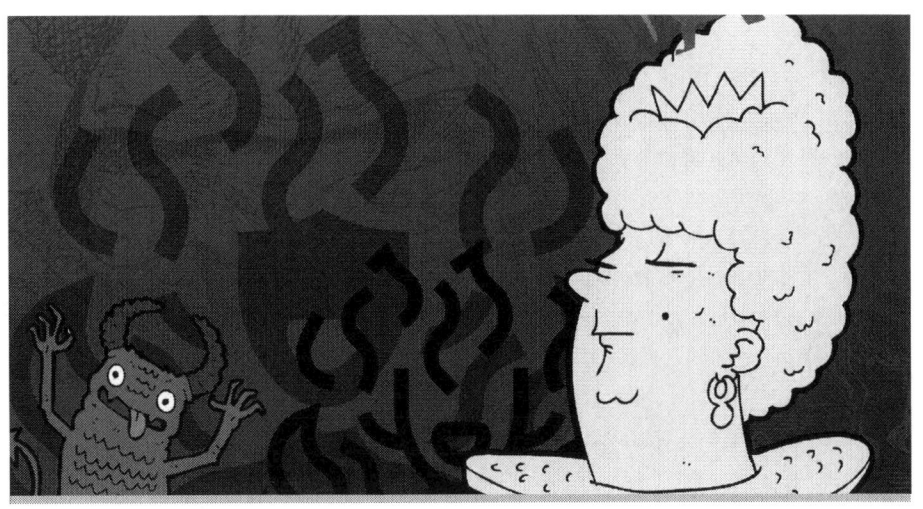

CHAPTER SIX

The Queen of Hearts

Grandiose narcissistic abusers demand immediate undivided attention and are insensible to effects of their direct demands of *entitlement* with others. You are not entitled to defy them. You are not entitled to your own muchness. You are not entitled to free will and be accepted by them. You are not entitled to behaviors that they deem embarrass or shame them publicly. You are not entitled to your own choices of clothing, your body, your value system...you are not entitled to the gift of free will. Obey or else... you are expendable. Their ability to retain a *grandiose sense of self* occurs with *self*-enhancement.

Grandiose narcissistic abusers are less sensitive than defenseless people, although they are dramatic *Red Queens* having temper tantrums. OFF with your head! The effects of their persistent emotional consequences are threats. They crave feeling validation of entitlement through expectations place on others while viewing others in contempt. No one is their equal. They are the only ones who are superior. No matter your age or stage of development, even as an adult...all you are in their eyes is a child to be controlled. You are '*diminutive and small.*' They feel they have a right even then to put their hands on you, and/or control you through punishment, where '"*silence is their validation.*'

Narcissistic abusers attempt to continue to manipulate you into feeling invalidated, so you doubt (1) the situation was really not as bad as you perceived and (2) to convince *others* who are their "chess pieces" (pawns) to move on their behalf. The *Queen of Hearts* they feel entitled to be manipulates the board of your life to place you in a defensiveness that send the message only they can move in any direction. Pawns carry out PR (public relations) on their behalf in the community to ensure their narrative of *their* self-image is *strictly* professed and adhered to. They will call you names and make public untrue accusations to turn others things they say are true that are not. THEY are pathological liars. They often believe their own narratives AND can convince others they are telling the truth about you! This is WHY it feels so overwhelming to go to court, to confront them, to find support from other friends and family members, to go to church pastors about abuse that is occurring right under their noses behind closed doors!

While the *Queen of Hearts* and *White Rabbit* narcissistic abuser combination screams OFF with your head in private, the community is under the impression of the *Queen of Hearts* as charming, caring, a *good* person, *incapable* of abuse, *generous* to others, *kind*, doubting the vehement cruelty they enforce of you when he/she does not get their way. They *fake* empathy. They *crave* admiration.

Narcissistic abusers have the ability to feign the reality of what they are doing to you so well you also doubt yourself and what reality you *know* to be true! They crave opportunities to ridicule you and accuse you falsely of things you would not or have not done. Then turn it back on you when you confront the lies...using phrases of shock and awe, "I would never say or do anything like that to you!" They cannot take responsibility for what they do to others.

Often, a quick *(fake)* apology holds attached blame and conditions such as, this is what you did *"but you...made me..."* do (blank). *"IF you would just, but...do I tell you to then, I wouldn't have to yell and scream and direct your childish ways then!"* Although we can all develop a situational need to consider *self* with boundaries...we all experience negative days, trauma affects our interactions with others. For the narcissistic abuser, they are *not* going through a situational phase even when they rant about it. For them, there is a persistent pattern of these behaviors over a lifetime and the situation is about *them*.

The effects on an individual who has suffered narcissistic abuse can be deadly, extremely debilitating, chronic, and individual recovery can be a complex process. The situations and interactions with them can be frightening and confusing and then they will drag YOUR support systems to them to use and manipulate you into their circle by showing favor and feigning a false sense of security and attachment. They are methodical planners and so you must be ten steps ahead knowing and recognizing what their behaviors mean...because they will use friends and family members t make sure they are on their side and their behaviors weren't really abusive. They will focus on your shortcomings and then when you finally speak out about the years of their malignant narcissistic abuse you may find yourself doubting YOUR reasons for your boundaries with a sense of maybe it wasn't that bad...he or she would never...he or she is so nice! They need others to idolize their goody two shoe identities! This gives them power to continue the cycle of shame and guilting you back into their circle of resources. They believe that whatever they need to do to get what they want is justified!

During childhood and adolescence, when our guardians, parents, people within our inner circles who are caregivers abuse their position of power we loose trust in who is considered 'over' or 'in authority' of us. Abuse derives from neglect, dismissal, emotional manipulations, ridicule, sexual abuse, physical abuse, oppressive situations, when we are scoffed at, laughed at in a negative context, bullied, controlled, objectified, our boundaries are breached without our permission or say so because to do so, to have boundaries assertively is deemed culturally as disrespectful, when we are seen and heard and not silent, we learn to dissociate from the world, turn inward, and what we develop rather is a threatened terrifying nightmare of existence we feel lost and abandoned within.

Our developing mind has aroused an unhealthy toxic ego, and we become unbalanced, stuck between the negative dialogue of lost child self, or critical parent critical caregiver critical self internally.

The message becomes encoded we are not safe. We decide others cannot be trusted to meet our needs. We learn to try and find solutions to outwit the manipulators, or we learn to blindly be manipulated without question in future relationships to be accepted and placate their narcissistic abuse. We learn we cannot engage our feelings, because to feel and to let that be made known is not safe. We disconnect with positive adaptations and solely identify with shame, guilt, whereas positive emotions are shut down. We set off on a destructive path because we have no positive identifiers encoded as truth statements any longer. We are on a continuum of devastation. Additionally, these maladaptive adaptations cause physical and brain damage due to the detrimental effects on (new books coming Buchanan 2022: 'Miss Amy G. Dala,' 'The Hippo Campus,' and 'Mr. Pre-Frontal Cortex).

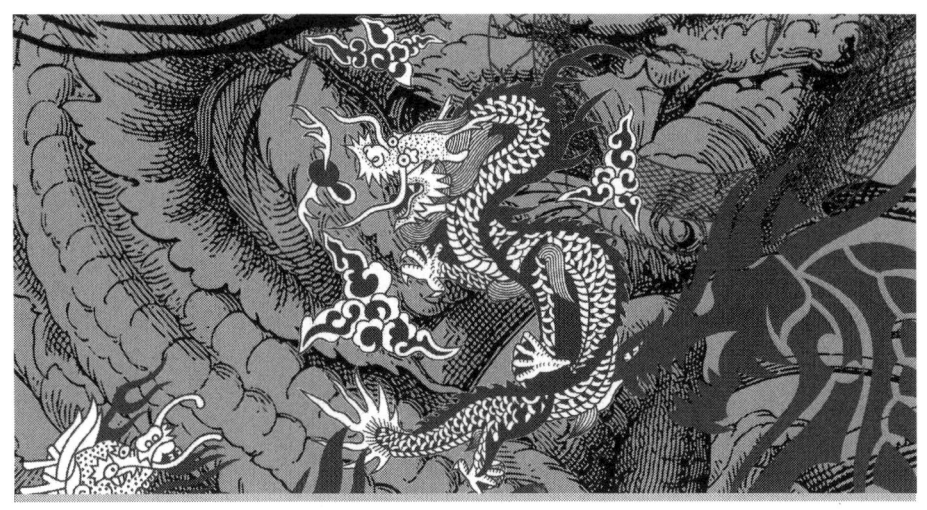

CHAPTER SEVEN

Jabberwocky

Lost In Twisted Wonderland Chased by *Time's* Jabberwocky, you feel lost, Alice. *'He jabbed me with his steal claws! He has bitten and split open my flesh with his grimacing jaws!'* Narcissistic abuse is brainwashing! It is intended to destroy your sense of self-worth and self-efficacy (*value*). You no longer feel like yourself...or you stop remembering what your unique MUCHNESS even really was! It is often impossible to recall when you were genuinely happy other than during the honeymoon phases of chronic control. Honeymoon phases are times when the Jabberwocky does not show his/her spots. They appear to be a time of interval of re-prieve, and often, these times are meant to strategically draw you back in to make you think they are choosing long term change and are ending their abusive ways. They seem 'nice' and this can last for a set time, and vary depending on how they are making your mind spin spin spin to draw you back in. *'How cheerfully he seems to grin How neatly spread his claws and chin, He welcomes innocent fishes in... With gentle smiling jaws within.'*

You struggle to recognize yourself in the looking glass with a Jabberwocky lurking right behind you. The reflection you see staring back at you is foreign...frightening. You may also feel as though you have turned into the jub-jub-jaberwocky yourself... because during the *honeymoon* phase they twist and turn things their way. Everything is your fault, *Dear Alice.* They will feign apologizing for their behaviors and attempt to (often very well) display sorrow and remorse, promising it won't happen again... they will change their ways.

This also motivates narcissistically abusive persons in that *validation* for them is something they crave, as long as they can control and dominate you. They need to be thanked and adored by others...they need supply. Getting supply means acting for even long intervals of time, in a helping caring manner, and boosts their public image. Narcissist's view others are objects and everyone in their social circle has a use...when you do not any longer participate in catering that, you are expendable, and this is when the shift occurs from the caring image to the abuser once again to gain control. *'Suddenly I hear the snarling coming back my way! I turn to run, to hide, to go away! The jub-jub jabberwocky at my back has now come!'* This pattern of ups and downs moving from one extreme to the next is traumatic for the brain to adapt to and process and encode, as the brain develops a fogginess in which category to store memories.

Traumatic stress from narcissistic abuse is associated with augmented levels of cortisol and norepinephrine responses to ensuing stressors. Since the normal human brain experiences fluctuations in structure and function across the lifespan from early childhood to late adulthood, during adolescence from age 7 to 17 years, there is a progressive increase in white matter (related to continuing myelination) and reduction in gray matter (related to neuronal pruning); while overall brain size stays the same (Bremmer, 2006). Maladaptively encoded memories create acute or chronic trauma. Trauma (post-traumatic stress disorder) is categorized by symptoms, including intrusive thoughts, hyperarousal, flashbacks, nightmares, and sleep disturbances, changes in memory and concentration, and startle responses.

Personal boundaries are frequently disregarded with the goal of molding and manipulating the adolescent to satisfy the parent's/partner's expectations (whether for perfection, image, or performance). Narcissistic parents are self-absorbed and grandiose. They are inflexible, and lack empathy required for child rearing and healthy attainment of the required stages of psychological development.

Grandiosity means to exhibit an unrealistic sense of superiority, characterized by a sustained view of self as better than others, expressed by condescendingly criticizing the adolescent, overinflating one's capability and belittling the adolescent as inferior; referring to a sense of personal uniqueness with a foundational belief that few other people have anything in common with, and can only be understood by a few, very superior individuals). *'To get attacked by the Jabberwocky who lurks all about. She grins wider and wider as I beg and plead for her to say which way, which way, do I go to stay safe!'*

The honeymoon phase is a twisting turning winding attack because they also manipulate you into having internal trust issues with yourself, and others…especially those closest to you who can clearly SEE the Jabberwocky for what they are. Or when those closest to you have been manipulated to see the Jabberwocky in you…and have been dupped into siding with the narcissist images of public niceness. *'The jub-jub jabberwocky at my back has won! There's no water to quench the hate that's burning inside. He has tasted my scream and gives in to pleasuring himself in my pain.'*

You feel responsible for your lostness. You feel hatred towards your muchness and the jabberwocky. Once you start breaking free of narcissistic abuse, the narcissist does not stop.

Behaviors often are exacerbated (in private) as you are sidelined and stressed even further feeling you have no true support system who believes in your experience. *'There's no need to run, he stalks and considers it fun. He plays the game with others you know... To make himself look innocent with you... the real trouble you know.'*

Narcissists will derail your goals and aspirations to sabotage you and talk down about you to others who want to give you favor to achieve your goals. They want you to *only* depend on them for your self-identity and to do otherwise is deeply intensely offensive to them, especially goals that do not align with *their* version of you under their control. They will seek to control *everything* about you: where you work, who you see, who you date, where you hang out, when you hang out, the social circles you are in, what clothes you are allowed to wear...your presentation to the community is a reflection on them, and they must match you to the dynamic they want to represent at all costs and especially pick fights or provoke you so that they can control you by unwarranted punishments, and in childhood, unwarranted grounding. They will play you like a fiddle putting you through a gauntlet of card soldiers scoffing at you and when you defy them because you decide to recognize the relationship and their presence and influence is unhealthy and toxic, you will struggle with feelings of inadequacy, unworthiness, and the belief that you did (*what they have told everyone else*) and deserved the treatment of you.

Your internal narrative becomes the ideology replaying that yells and screams at you that there is something *wrong* with you, and *nothing* wrong with what they did to you in their abuse of you. You are inherently wrong in defying them. Period. You wonder why you were not loved unconditionally...because they used their powers in such malevolent ways. You struggle with low self-esteem and believe the narcissistic abuser *would have* treated you better had you done what they said when they said it. *'There is no help coming. He locked the gate.'* This level of abusive stress results in acute and chronic alterations of neurochemical systems and specific brain regions. These changes result in long-term variations in brain circuits involved in our stress response (Bremmer,

2006). You have trouble focusing on your goals and dreams and aspirations the narcissist *made you* or *forced you* to give up on when it did not fit *their* narrative of their ability to control you. THEY require your submission AND the muchness of your mind Alice!

After narcissistic abuse, you are stressed about what happened to you. Yes, hindsight comes at you like a shuffled card deck, displaying faces of memories of events and you find it difficult to shut off your brain at night to just rest. *'There are only flamingos to swing ... and hedgehogs to roll past my feet.'* When you do rest nightmares take hold, and can haunt you for days, weeks, and even years afterwards. He has trapped you in time and due to this level of chronic stress, it is difficult to concentrate on work, watching television, performing everyday activities you once enjoyed. This is because of the surge of stress hormones affecting the hippocampus region post trauma. It is common to undergo mood swings, irritability, numbness, emotionless, on a robotic mode. You can experience depersonalization where it seems everything around you is not accurate. You feel outside of your own body, and nothing is real (derealization), or both. You experience panic and experience separation anxiety and disorientation because you are not with the narcissistic abuser, extreme fear and anxiety in new relationships with new people. *'In the endless game should you dare try to sneak away, He will find you and snare you open with a gash of his teeth!'*

During adolescence and throughout adulthood, the brain undergoes pruning, and many of the most significant changes in the frontal cortex and parietal cortex occur throughout adolescence into young adulthood. Pruning allows the overpopulation of neurons and synaptic connections to be regulated. We lose what we do not need; however, this is also negative. During, for example, narcissistic abuse in childhood due to childhood stressors, too much pruning can occur due to toxicity in the neuronal connections and circuitry in the hippocampus (storing of memories), the corpus collosum (linking left and right brain hemispheres), and the prefrontal cortex. This effects decision making abilities, self-regulation, attention, emotional regulation, positive adaptive thought encoding, and behaviors. Adversity changes the way the brain prunes adaptive or maladaptive responses.

It is my hypothesis clinically, that since brain regions associated with trauma include the hippocampus, amygdala, and medial prefrontal cortex, when from narcissistic abuse occurs during adolescence these occurrences lessen positive resiliency and increase risk for survivors developing chronic PTSD. This predisposes us to being in traumatizing abusive situations in the future. Cortisol and norepinephrine are two (of many) neurochemical systems critical in our stress response. These neurochemicals interact with additional compounds in our brain to referee fear-related (at times, unnecessary) physiological processes, and memories. Therefore, they become encoded into our memory bank like files of unfinished homework. We continue to replay events with triggers and reminders from the rabbit hole.

What is experienced as a result are panic attacks, anxiety, depression, physical symptoms such as headaches, migraines, body aches, stomachaches, cognitive issues, loss of self-worth, trouble making decisions, confusion, feeling stuck. This is exacerbated when narcissistic abuser *hoovers* (the term for acting nice like a vacuum cleaner) merely for the purpose of being able to suck you back in. They will call, email, or contact you in their attempts to manipulate you back into *their circle* or *feeling sorry* for whatever they are experiencing or professing they are going through. They count on and play on your empathy to transform it into sympathy and feeling sorry for them to justify and ignore their pervasive pattern of behaviors and abuse. (The question is not *if* they attempt to contact you, but *when* and how much they will be allowed to violate your boundaries). They NEED to keep you or get you back into being *trapped* in their cycle. They NEED you to stay or jump back into their rabbit holes to become lost again in Twisted Wonderland! They are master manipulators. 'They studied... and knew I wanted to just stay safe... They studied... and knew the pains of my past I had not yet escaped.'

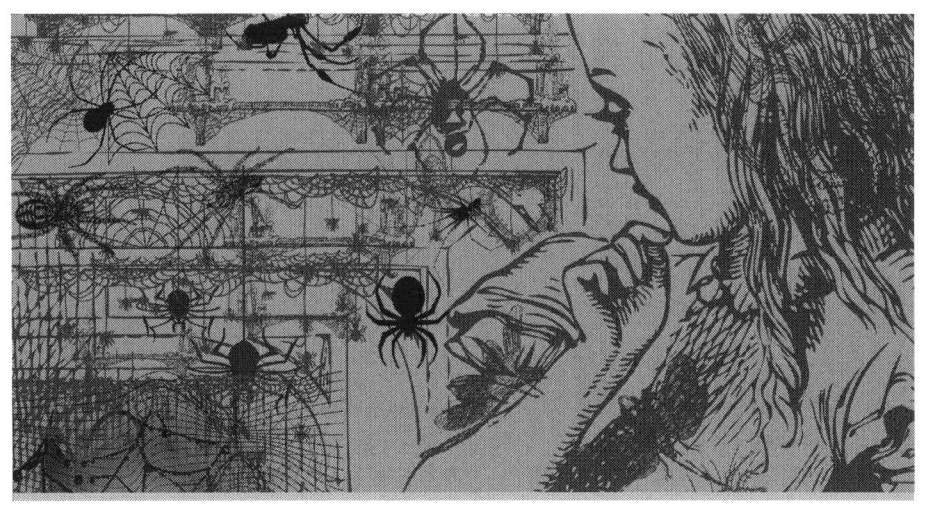

CHAPTER EIGHT

The Trap

Behaviors of fight, flight, or freeze occur during our brain's response to what it perceives as emotional and psychological torture. This continuous overload of events our brain perceives as life threatening become negative stress associated with toxic shifting alterations in various stages of our natural development. This occurs alongside hippocampal adjustments, and significantly lowers resiliency abilities due to exposures of: (1) repeated anguish, included nutritional deficiencies common with comorbid abuse; (2) physical punishment (experiencing repeated flight/fight/freeze dopaminergic alternations); (3) severe beatings or threats to one's life (as the brain perceives during emotional and psychological abuse), and (4): horrendous mental and psychological tortures.

The overall stress adrenal and dopaminergic activations become *stunted*, under-developed and severe enough during various vulnerable stages of development to develop psychological difficulties following traumatic events. We develop PTSD from narcissistic abuse through exposures to ongoing traumas (each maladaptively encoded event) that are *not* normal (*adjustment disorder* is a psychological response to a *common stressor* and occurs due to a change in everyday life, not ongoing life-threatening events as the brain perceives them to be, or exposure to an actual or threatened serious events). *'They set up a trap within your heart and mind... and you give place to their destruction in kind.'*

Adjustment disorder is the *mildest* result of maladaptively encoded traumatic events that are common stressors. PTSD is intrusive and debilitating; wherein, a pathological memory has formed at the center of the brain and body response. With PTSD you find it difficult to trust others. *'Trust is hard to find in this place.'* This leaks into your present and future relationships when not healed and worked through, because we have to deprogram these encoded repetitive maladaptive (brainwashed) patterns of self-destruction. *'You seek to allow them to break me down, to kill, steal and destroy'*

It is easy to wonder lost wondering if everyone is as mad as the abuser, if everyone is stuck in teatime, if everyone is untrustworthy. It can become difficult for others to be honest with you, because the trauma has a maladaptive affect of becoming hypervigilant to criticism and being overly sensitive to judgement from others due to the encoded fears of being betrayed. *'It's not safe to feel safe it's not okay to feel okay.'*

Narcissistic abuse may also create a negative cycle of people pleasing and feelings of panic and fear over perceived abandonment with insecure attachment issues shadowing behind you like a jabberwocky. Because you had to walk on eggshells for so long, and being brainwashed into people pleasing is a hard cycle to break because of the encoded constant need to rescue others and wear *their* emotional baggage. Everything was *your fault*, remember, Alice? You feel you need to be constantly overaccommodating to gain approval to encourage others to like you. This is because the narcissistic abuse left you feeling alone and abandoned with your support circle growing smaller and smaller as the narcissist was able to deceive others with the constant nice person routine and community PR. *'Please him at all costs, you're trapped in his madness. You belong to this place filled with hate filled sadness.'*

You had to learn to keep your muchness to yourself...and so you struggle with emotional regulation and expressing your thoughts and due to underlying fear of being judged and ridiculed. You had to keep your muchness, Alice, contained within a bottle...you had to shrink down your size to be smaller to appease the abuser. You learned to punish yourself, *stupid girl*, for having thoughts of being intelligent and smart, not *trouble*, but *valuable*... and you feel at fault for their bad behaviors towards you. Therefore, you have or continue to, seek self-destructive behaviors. When we have no control we seek what we can control...and so addictions are common....they provide a way to try and numb the emotional pain. *'Broken I am I want to go away. I want to disappear like a ghost, just away.'*

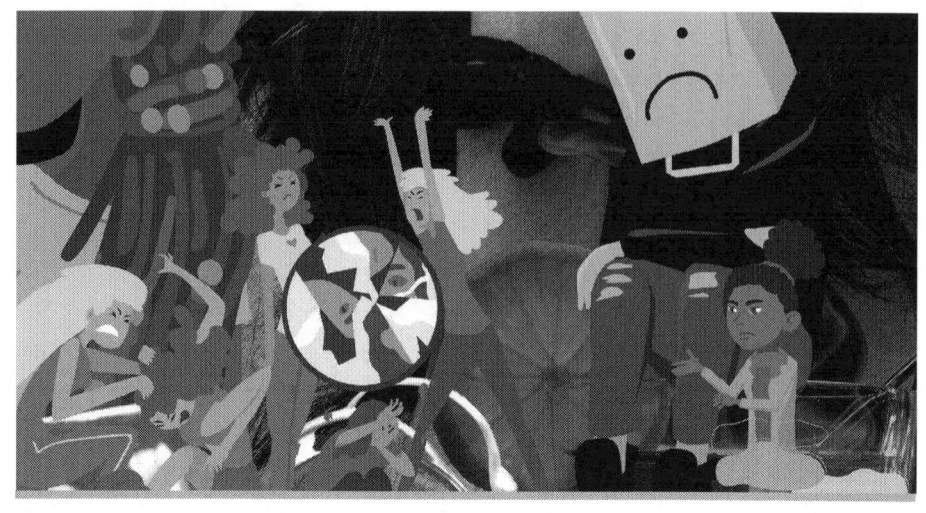

CHAPTER NINE

A Mad Tea Party

Victims of narcissistic abuse seem uncertain of themselves and can feel the need to constantly seek clarification they have not made a mistake or misheard. As a reactive adaptation to narcissistic abuse, this is because the narcissistic person constantly finger-points and shifts blame to you for encoding the negative cognition of responsibility for their ups and downs in the relationship and in their own psyche. In these types of twisted relationships, there are non-existent boundaries. They will come into the room of your personal space when they want to, do what they want to, everything is in their control, their power. Everything is their property. There is no escape. They berate and browbeat you they are always right. Their way or the highway. Period. No discussion.

You find yourself constantly put on edge and dumped on, feeling an immense sense of overpowering forced to accept responsibility for things you did not do or say. Every response is a provoking response. Every defense or healthy assertive boundary is disrespect. This borrowed humiliation and shame is what the narcissist intends for you to accept from them. It is a reflection of their own internal unfelt core of shame. *'No matter the cost, dear Alice in this garden of memory, Ignore these demons that roam this sky! This palace of dreams, pretend you are mad too and it won't feel like it seems!'*

You may begin to slowly realize the realities and borders between yourself and others is not only blurred but missing, toxic, unhealthy. However, it can feel overwhelming and confusing to make the brain deprogram the adaptive response that you are not responsible for someone else's behaviors towards you, or what they chose to do as a result of their rage at losing control over you, or you no longer choosing their chaos...the thinking and feeling of being constantly scolded for behaving, thinking and feeling is out of control. *'You're nothing but what he wants you to be... His blind fury is that of red...quick to sentence you to emotional and psychological death.'*

Although it is difficult to accept, unconsciously, the narcissistic personality person does know how to manipulate in such a way to re-program you to feel you have a divided and conquered mind. *'You, Twisted Alice, you sit there in vain! You act like you don't want me! So where do I stay? In this dark dark road in this tea-party of madness.'* You are supposed to be their most vulnerable and susceptible target who will not be able to identify the confusion caused by the abusive technique 'gaslighting.' *'Distressing unresolved memories will prevail! I say!'* Gaslighting is psychological abuse used by narcissistic abusers and the tool is intended to inject confusion and anxiety in you as the target to the point you no longer trust you *own* memory, *perception*, or *judgment*. *'Eventually this madness will drive who you are 'supposed to be away.'*

With gas lighting, the target...you...initially notices something happens and the something that happens is odd, and at the same time, you deny the truth and do not believe it. You attempt to fight the manipulation and become also confused by being called names or told you are: *'Just Too sensitive', 'Crazy', 'Imagining things'* and the narcissist flat out DENIES saying (or doing) *anything* hurtful. 'You did that to yourself' (after they hit you).

Gradually, you learn not to trust your own perception and begin doubting yourself...and another added bonus...they also gaslight YOUR other support networks...that PR image thing again, Dear Alice, where they convince others they could not possibly do those things, and even to deny them being a witness to such horrors without *your* provocation. Broken and unable to trust yourself (and others) you isolate further. You now doubt *everything* about yourself: your thoughts, opinions, values, ideas, ideals, and your MUCHNESS that makes you unique. *'I'm drained from trying to shield! It leaks out! It looks like I hate everything when I freak out!'* You become dependent on the narcissist for *their* perception of reality, or you become targeted by their onslaught of revenge tactic when you refuse to accept their control. *'Succumb Twisted Alice, my dear, here sit sit...'* What they want to succeed at is you screaming internally *'You act like you don't want me! So where do I stay'* And they will say with their actions, *'In this dark dark road in this tea-party of madness.'*

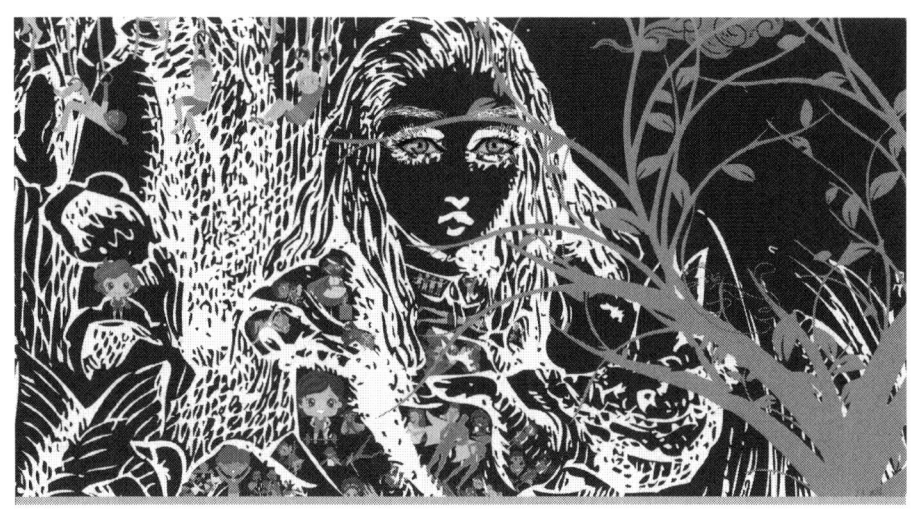

CHAPTER TEN

The Queen's Gambit

In chess, the opening that starts with the moves, is the *Queen's Gambit.* It is the oldest opening in chess. In the Queen's Gambit, White appears to sacrifice one the pawns...the C pawn. It seems to be a contradiction in chess play because Black cannot hold the pawn without encountering a disadvantage. It is a positional play in strategy, allowing for gaining and exploiting for small advantages rather than larger more apparent advantages of position and requires calculating immediate tactics. *'I feel so used. I feel so alone; I feel the darkening madness.'* It is a calculated symmetrical move in chess, purposeful to sacrifice a *'pawn'* to gain leverage, or control of the board. It provides with better success at winning the game.

In early stages of chess, control of the center of the board is vital and places your opposition unawares, on defense, and pressured by an opponent. When played currently, the Queen's Gambit forces Black to spend the game responding to threats rather than being able to think through and strategize an opposition. '*I am trying so hard to ignore the pain knocking and rap rap rapping at my door.*' What occurs when a narcissistic abuser plays a Queen's Gambit in the opening of the relationship is setting the stage for you to be on defense, giving him/her opportunity to exchange his/her wing pawn to gain control of your center of being...YOUR muchness. It is the oldest opening move in chess history...trading something of value to gain leverage.

The reasoning? Dear Alice...the Queen in terms of RAW power is the MOST powerful piece in chess, and in all creation! You, *Dear Alice*, are created to have such a long range of talents, gifts...you are able to move in multiple directions, multi-task, help to create and carry life within you! We are the bringers of Life Himself! We were never an after-thought of creation but the first thought of the Deliverance of the One Who Sacrifices His own Life for us!

In chess, a Queen can control up to a total of 28 squares on the board...and a king, although the right one who is not an unhealthy toxic narcissistic abuser, only controls a total of 9 squares from the center of the board. The Queen is the most powerful chess piece because she is able to move any number of squares. She can move horizontally, vertically, diagonally. She can combine her strength with her community and make it stronger! Pawns can be promoted and raised up to become Queens. She alone is worth 9 pawns! This in chess terms, means SHE is stronger than a rook AND a Bishop put together!

A QUEEN is strongest when the chess board is open and the enemy *king* is poorly defended. SHE is stronger in closed positions. Narcissistic abusers are attracted to strong, confident, self-assured women because of their traits of grandiosity and confidence being a mask of deep insecurity, and this is also why narcissistically abusive parents and guardians, likewise, are so vehemently in opposition and violent with children (especially female children) who are considered by the narcissistic parent to be obstinate, disrespectful, disobedient, noncontrollable.

Narcissistic abusers utilize a mask of self confidence and assurance portraying the image of someone who will provide strength, and the ability to manage any situation. They become what the woman wants, for a time...or portray themselves as the perfect parent. The charade of authenticity occurs until the relationship is solidified and they reveal their true personality (behind closed doors as the image is still to protected at all costs).

Since narcissists want to feel real empathy, and cannot, and want to be kind, and do not, they see a strong woman as a conquest to be provided with a sense of worthiness at the cost of your own. Their power and domination over you provide them with a sense of superiority and authority. That power gives them a sense of twisted pleasure. *'You say I shouldn't be so 'me,' My muchness must stay away I must be Twisted Alice to survive forever from this day!'*

Mr. Mrs. Perfect pushes boundaries and plays on your empathy through manipulation blaming and attempts to backhand compliment insult you also shift's blame on you through shaming and doing what they want to do. They play the victim when things do not go their way and will prioritize their needs above your own...and use what you are protective over as a weapon. Your emotions, your safe space, your children, your independence, your family and friends, your alone time. They are highly sensitive to any form of criticism of themselves; however, will run you through the chopping block screaming *'Off with her head That Alice is too much! She's so high and mighty in her confidence, I'll destroy it at once!'* They demand you put THEM first...above yourself and call your needs selfish when you question their domineering authority. They will call you ungrateful and spoiled, even when you arc not that kind of person. They need someone who makes them look good. The more accomplished and good looking you are, the more your MUCHNESS brains brawn and beauty get his twisted ego. However, a narcissistic abuser will not tolerate a woman who is stubborn in her muchness.

Self-confidence and stubbornness are traits they cannot handle. However, he may twist the game and predicate on your emotional side as they need constant attention and emotional validation at all costs...your muchness, your family, your children, you! Narcissistic abusers monopolize relationships, and they are not willing to sustain more than feigned compromises. They drive you to become low in harm avoidance and extremely high in cooperation and giving in to their twisted games or engaging in their demands and avoiding conflict allows them to be provided empathy and attention. *'I think she must learn how to mind. Just cut off her head...'*

The narcissistic abuser will not take responsibility or accountability for their actions...it is always someone else's fault who made them...and the love-bombing, Dear Alice, is their Queen's Gambit, intended to take you off guard and unsure, and to be on alert but confused and on edge; yet defensive and confused. *'At least THEN she won't bother me with her emotional mind! CUT OFF HER BLASTED HEAD! She always pretends like she's hurting inside! She screams and fights back, how dare she defy!'* They demand someone to worship them and make them look good without them doing the self-efforts for genuine improvement. Since he needs someone loyal and strong he can count on to take care of him, who provides empathy to attend to the childlike needs they display, who demand you to stroke their ego...Dear Alice, as a Queen, they are a formidable enemy. He needs to impress you to pull of his Queen's Gambit. *'You Alice, this muchness is a thing of the past! There's no future for you outside of this wonderland I have amassed!*

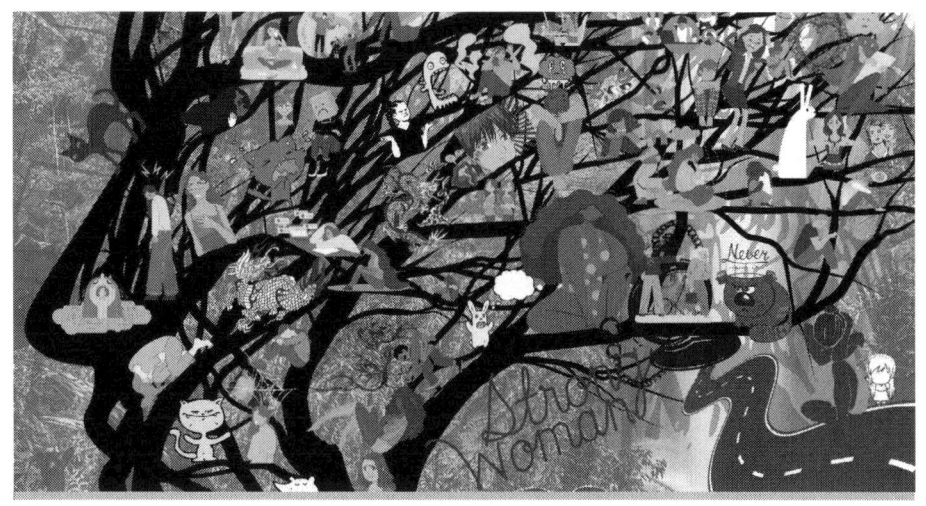

CHAPTER ELEVEN

Twisted Alice

There is a biological connection between narcissistic abusers and aggression. Aggression, at the right times, when it is healthy can be adaptive. However, when not used as a weapon, is intended to harm. There is more than one type of aggression in developmental psychology. Even with various differences in research, most agree to predatory aggression and affective aggression. Predatory aggression in narcissistic abuse is purposeful. It's intention is a premeditated unprovoked attack, is cold, and emotionless. Affective aggression is impulsiveness within emotional arousal, instrumental. Instrumental for the narcissistic abuser results in a gain for the abuser...and are actions they do purposely to intimidate and frighten you. Their anger and rage can be frightening. It is terrorizing to both children and as an adult woman.

Narcissistic abusers who are parents lack empathy, exploit children for their own agendas, and are improbable to pursue long term treatment or change for the long term, destructive behaviors against their children, even into adulthood (Kacel, Ennis, & Pereira, 2017). Children suffer severe psychological maltreatment when parents employ behaviors like bullying, terrorizing, coercive control, insults, demands, and threats against them or their safe places and safe people to keep them compliant. These extremes against Dear Alice's produce unhealthy toxic results. These behaviors place children of narcissistic parent(s) at risk for suicidality, low self-esteem, depression, self-harm, substance abuse, attachment disorders, complex PTSD, and leads to symptoms children display who have been physically and sexually abused (Gibson, 2016; Schwartz, 2016; Spinazzola et al., 2014, Walker, 2013). *'I'm lost in your folly! I can't take any more of this unrelenting madness! I'm just a Mock Turtle I always feel sadness!'*

The narcissistic abuser parent or person may *appear* to make a request. However, it is a demand. When you set a healthy assertive boundary and say no to the request that compromises your safety, they continue to apply increased pressure and threaten consequences to attempt to get you to concede to them. When you continue to refuse, especially when they are being controlling and overtly harsh and demanding, and demeaning to you, they will punish you with their sulking, passive-aggressive arguments, a rage attack, withholding something of value they have already promised you, and threat violence or enact sabotage against the safe persons you have connected to who are healthy for you and enabling you to cope with them. This is emotional extortion.

The narcissistically abusive person or parent(s) use fear, guilt, and obligations to arouse guilt that manipulates us to give into *their* desires at the expense of our own basic needs and rights. We each have been gifted FREE WILL by our Creator Himself. We are not the property of any person. We are not obligated to live for anyone else other than our choices in our faith. For me, Jesus

Christ...not who blank ever. I chose Him, He chose me. HE is healthy and does not obligate, manipulate, or demean. He does not need to guilt or instill obligatory guilt and unhealthy fear through intimidation.

The narcissistic abuser drills it into you through his/her fits of rage and violence to teach you to walk on eggshells around them *or* there will be consequences. You need to *'be quiet.'* Their consequences are implanting a fear of a reaction, caution when you do or say something only to have words are twisted up on you. You feel you must choose your words carefully and avoid discussing certain topics to offend them...because they are always right and explosive when you have a different opinion. You try to avoid conflict; however, they crave your adoration, command your attention, and dominate the conversation with their overbearingness. They *'never'* seem to listen to you...or hear your plight against their rage. *'I've changed so much...several times since we met. I'm so sick of trying to explain myself. I followed this rabbit and got lost trying to solve this puzzle of who I am.'* However, what they are really doing is to provoke your amygdala to stay alert because you are hypervigilant in knowing when their next attack will come... and how strong and how rageful it will be. They strive to keep you in a state of heightened anxiety and fear to bend you to staying in the emotional prison or Twisted Wonderland. *'This isn't a fairytale how will this wonderland END!'*

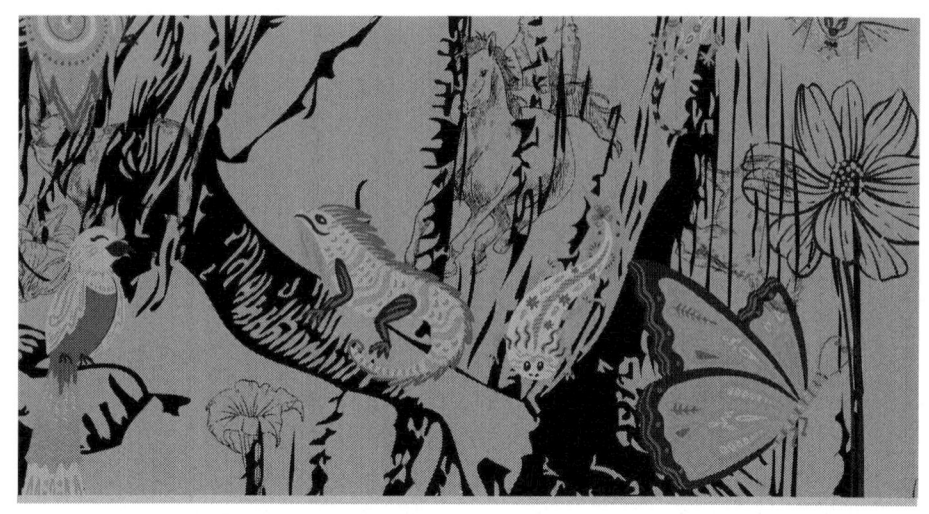

CHAPTER TWELVE

The Real Alice

King David praised in his awareness that we are each fearfully and wonderfully made! (Psalms 139:14).   No matter your faith or religious connection, this truth is an assertively loving self-cognition! In Psalms (the book of poems), David is the Hebrew Third King of the United Monarchy of Israel. It is important for him to share with others as King that God created us each UNIQUE! We each have a *right* under His creation to our *autonomy* even when narcissistically abusive toxic parents disagree with your choices.

We do not owe someone an explanation for our choices about our career, love life, or children we choose to have. We are not responsible for *their* perception of their social image. However, with a narcissistic parent and a narcissistic person, *their* image is all that matters. They expect you to bend your created muchness to fit THEIR box and dynamic of who *they* think you should be. It has nothing to do with you...everything to do with them.

You should not question, according to their perception, even their abuse of you, or assertively tell them please stop, I will not be treated or hit. I do not want to be hit. To speak up, even in healthy ways is...the cloak term used by narcissistic parents '*disrespectful*.' To the narcissist, healthy assertive boundaries ARE 'disrespectful' AND reality, Dear Alice's, healthy assertive adaptive boundaries do not make them wrong.

The narcissist parent will not let you live it down when you stand up to their unhealthy abusive manipulation. They will not accept the word no when they are in the wrong and are highly and often uncontrollably abusive. They do not perceive *their* actions and control are abusive. They have a pervasive pattern of the driving need to be out of control in their control of others.

A parent who is healthy can want to genuinely support you to be your best self, and to accomplish your goals...a narcissistic parent or person only wants for you to live in their box of what they deem for you. Your unique gifts, talents, temperament... that is expendable when it is in contradictory to their image. Another tool used against you to ensure compliance at all costs, is to control you through unwarranted shame, belittlement, and demeaning actions towards you. Nitpicking, shaming, and then false compliments to keep you off track are unnerving. Especially when you have siblings. Their favorite tools for control to keep you in line is to teach you through subservience to walk on eggshells and appease them.

Narcissistically abusive parents spend a great deal of conversation throughout siblings' lifetimes comparing each child to other siblings and peers to diminish you. They need you to act as the scapegoated child (even as an adult) to fight for *their* approval and attention. Therefore, they provoke you into feeling *less than*. '*Perpetually trapped in the mirrored image in a glass house. This rude-*

ness is more than I can possibly bear. I am confused and confuzzled. I don't know how I even got here! Can't I just change my size and get the hell out of here! Can't I just get the key to escape this nightmare!' However, *'Dear Alice, it's me, the true you inside...Not the Twisted Alice, the Real Alice...The one who been hiding while you're dying inside. Don't throw me away just because you feel overwhelmed today.'*

In developmental psychology, a useful trick regarding awareness of our attention, is called the *Cheshire Cat* effect. While having a friend stand in front of you, hold a mirror in your LEFT hand and block your right eye's view of your friend's face, but NOT his/her left eye. Now hold your right hand so you can see your hand in the mirror (and standing in the corner of a room with blank walls on both sides works best). Your hand, and your friends face will appear in the same position, and your friends face, or part of his/her face will...disappear! When you hold your hand steady, you will see your friends face again through your own transparent hand. Move your hand slightly and his/her face disappears again. You can leave your friend only with a Cheshire Cat grin.

Why does this happen? Your brain sends information from your eyes that are conflicted of two objects in the same position. Binocular rivalry is the result. The brain attends to one stimulus for a time and then switches to the other. Attention switches when your friends face or head, move. *Dear Alice's...*THIS is what your brain has done to YOU in your traumas of surviving narcissistic abuse. Narcissists *cause* relational problems and predicate on those who are strong, loyal, have strong levels of empathy, who are caretakers, and who have the temperament gifts of the servant's heart.

Their struggles with superiority and self-loathing simultaneously cause you to focus on what is directly in front of you to survive...and your muchness, like the Cheshire Cat effect...seems to disappear. They think about other people as objects to and use you for selfish gain through their systematic patterns of emotional, psychological abuse consisting of neglect, rejection, oppression, degradation, misogyny (or misandry), cruelty, and even physical abuse when they lose their tempers. What you're giving to them, which is your all, is not enough for that person AND it never will be.

There is always going to be a persistent pervasive pattern of unhealthy toxic demands cloaked in smoke and mirrors to force you to remain focused on them and their needs, and not you... YOU are the cost. That YOU is also the Cheshire Cat effect, the muchness of the True Alice, the Real Alice that is crying and dying inside who seems to have just faded away. Like a ghost, just away.

A narcissistic abuser will not be content with what they have, or who you are. They will not accept your defiance. They have a compulsion to pervasively require *more*. Until your sense of self-worth is reduced to worthlessness because the narcissist is inept of being satisfied or reciprocal when he/she steals your muchness from you. This is when the narcissist abandons you because you have nothing to offer them further. You are used up and he/she demands new supply of admiration and mental energy. This is why they often MOVE areas and jobs so much in their lifetime...they need new public supply. They require you to be willing to give without needing anything REAL in return, especially from yourself.

This erosion of your *True Alice*, the *Real Alice's* value by the narcissistic abuser does occur overnight but is a deceptive, ongoing, and intention deterioration that also gradually trauma bonds you to them so that you feel you cannot leave, and your muchness, like the friend in the experiment standing physically in front of you, is gone...hiding, while you are dying inside. *'That muchness of you Alice, you're the only one, you know. All that grit and that temper is to keep you fighting for me. You'll see I will show you... when you let me be free!'*

You have been triangulated and played against others... your siblings and your cousins, your nephews, and nieces. You have found yourself vying for the narcissist's attention and rewards. You have been gaslighted and lied to. Your realities have been dismissed. For a time, you were not okay with trusting your own judgement and perceptions of reality. You have been demeaned and shamed. When you have been great at something (such as writing, sports, art, music) behind closed doors you were on the receiving end of their jealousy and threats...those outlets that are healthy are the first valuable items targeted to gain control and keep it...always dangling carrots over your head. In public audience, however, the same narcissistic parent has held YOUR talents up as a source of pride (and although HEALTHY parents offer this valuable praise) for the narcissistic parent it was not about you, but about them. A way to place the attention on themselves. You have been trapped at the table of teatime after teatime.

You have been criticized and idealized, Dear Alice's. You have been showered with love bombing (rewards for compliance and as supply). You have been stuck in Time's loop running in circles that repeat. You, like the original Alice, have been traversing through Wonderland initially as a child, walking, walking, walking, spinning, spinning, spinning into your adulthood. You were assigned a role you never signed up for. You were engaged as the scapegoat of the family, hero golden child, or invisible child. You either did it all wrong, or nothing wrong one day and the were used and compared to and manipulated by the narcistic parent to keep you spinning by suddenly switching roles to gain your favor and draw you back in the next. You were placed in a game of croquet 'with hedgehogs at your feet and flamingoes to swing' expecting to be placed in your voluntold role of the primary adored child while living often short term in awe of your narcissistically abusive and manipulative parent. You were forced to subjugate your needs (by Time and the Cheshire Cat) to keep the peace and placate Time's rage. Walking on swift feet and soft flowers became your norm. As you grew, Dear Alice's, you may have attracted other Time's into your loops, but Dear Alice, you do not have to stay in a Twisted Wonderland with the March Hare's, court jesters, or dormouse's. You do not have to choose to keep learning how to mind. You do not have to give up your muchness to Time!

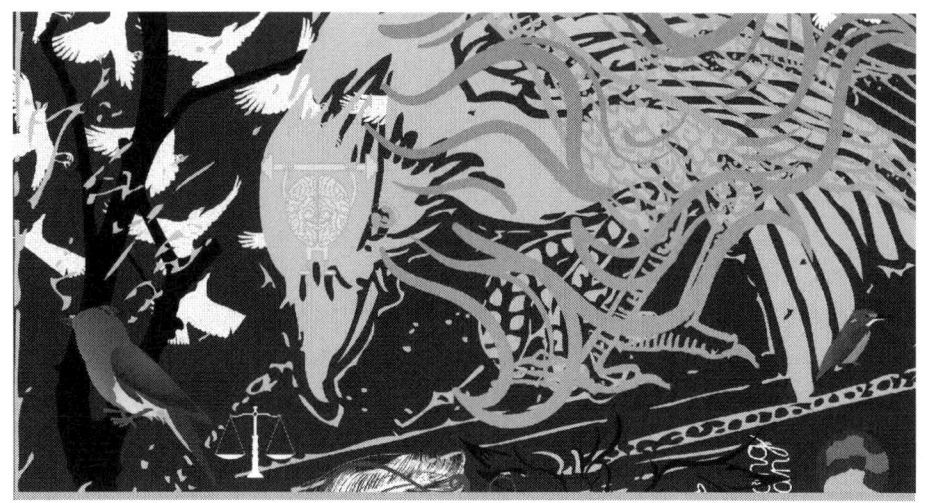

CHAPTER THIRTEEN

Who Stole the Muchness Alice's?

Freedom of Twisted Wonderland

Narcissistic abuse has the power to crush you irreparably, to kill, steal, destroy you, and it does not have to. YOU can take your power back. YOU can find your own unique MUCHNESS, Dear Alice's. It takes healthy development and therapeutic re-programming of positive brain body adaptations within nature and nurture to conquer residual effects of narcissistic abuse in trauma therapy. When we are no longer in a relationship that treats us as objects but are supported as persons who are individually created with unique temperament blends strengths and weaknesses, with healthy connections, growing together in healthy ways, we can *therapeutically* learn to process traumas, reprocess the brain and bodies negative affect, and develop positive self-awareness to heal. (In therapy).

Our fears can be abated, and we are therefore, restored. We can work through the mirrors of little Alice's in our own mental timelines to allow them EACH to have a voice, be recognized, healed, and validated in their experiences. (I use this original analogy in EMDR with my patients). *'She will know her value and her worth and she is fearless.'*

Rather than feeling like a piece being played on a chess board, we become chess masters of our own lives. We can reconnect with our True Alice, True Self inside. We can choose to halt the intergenerational curses from narcissistic abuse and trauma from our children repeating the patterns. The longer we reside in a threatening and abusive environment, the deeper we fall into the rabbit hole of Twisted Wonderland, the deeper our sense of healthy self-efficacy will devolve from a balanced ego exacerbating the fragility of our experiences. Behind the narcissistic abuser, is a hidden destructive jub-jub-jaberwocky locked within our internal dialogue.

We can learn to have the power to slay that version mentally and come out of the deepest darkest parts of the waking nightmares of Twisted Wonderland. We can choose not to allow another abuser into our lives and use healthy boundaries for the ones we feel we cannot fully escape from physically. We have the power to not continue to feel lost. We have the power to learn who we are, fearfully and wonderfully made. I do encourage you to do so with a good therapist.

In adulthood, *Dear Alice*, your size does not always protect you. Their pervasive pattern of destruction can have a lasting effect and cause a regression into childhood states of fear, shame, and terror, because of the provocation of the amygdala, hippocampal, prefrontal cortex fight/flight/freeze responses with maladaptively encoded unresolved events in the neural network. One variant to your size, is as an adult, you may choose your boundaries, your MUCHNESS, your own choices of self-care and a healthy boundary for many Dear Alice's is to limit contact with parents as you heal.

It takes energy to heal from betrayal, heartbreak, gaslighting, and losses from narcissistic abuse. If you are struggling, healing is important. Therapy helps you to be able to recognize, feel, deal with, sit with, and accept your feelings. At Acorns n Bones OMC, I teach clients our clinical model and AnBOMC tagline that therapy also educates you so you can *'Get Up, Be Raised Up'* in knowledge, therapy provides you with a support group and community with understanding and validation, and therapy teaches you the value and how to's of SELF care and how to *'Grow!'*

'One day you'll soar on wings of eagles of a Griffin. You'll know your value and worth and leave this abuse behind...' It is not easy, because you will hurt so much inside. The narcissistic abuser's tools have a toll... the shame, trauma, and lack of autonomy keep you trapped in the toxic relationship and keep the little Alice's trapped in their timeline of twistedness screaming. Narcissists are master manipulators and are able to disguise manipulation as love, passion, and great concern for other people and their relationship. They are good at lying and fool many people, even licensed therapists (which is why I went and earned Summa cum laude on a fourth Master of Science Forensic Psychology degree studying personality disorders). When their lies are exposed, they continue to tell lies to gaslight others attempting to convince them that they are wrong about their perceptions and assumptions.

Gaslighting has been used against you, Real Alice's, to deliberately cause you to believe *you* are crazy and have imagined the abusive actions they have committed against you to control and confuse you and others. They have spent significant time, Dear Alice's, comparing himself/herself to others to paint their life and personhood as superior to everyone else. You and your muchness, Dear Alice's, must mean nothing UNLESS it serves THEIR image and makes them look good! However, the fear intimidating and hypervigilance, Dear Alice's, you feel out of nowhere are because they have spent considerable time provoking and terrorizing you. Their use of angry outbursts and fearful rage was another way to manipulate you. When they puffed up their *chest*, got into your face, balled up their fists at their sides and postured to get ready to attack you...your brain encoded all of that. Their threatening physical violence, fear tactics, and intimidation to get what they want and to make you conform to their wishes can carry over into your everyday lives with yourself, with your children, and with your spouse.

You get your muchness BACK, Dear Alice's, by healing from the events of the traumas and the maladaptively encoded self-thoughts that came with their abusive programming. For me, God moved me 'far far away...' and He gave *me* time to heal, from *Time* the abuser(s). I had to accept that I needed therapy to break from the cycle of traumatic responses that had taken over *my* muchness.

The reality, Dear Alice's is that Time does not know how to really love you and that is not something you can teach them. They will tell you they do, and believe they do; however, it can only be transactional and conditional. They do not know how to not attach conditions because narcissism is a *pervasive condition* of low empathy, inter and intrapersonal exploitations, and entitlement not deeply felt love even when it looks convincing. Their feelings are changeable and shallow. They do not have the ability to place others best interests first, only what they perceive to be the best interests THEY have for others unless they are gaining supply from the appearances of caring-ness. They PRETEND. They pretend to keep up this false persona projected to the outside world. They cannot tolerate their feelings of unworthiness and inadequacies, and Dear Alice's, this is what is projected onto you to absorb. *"You will absorb all of this madness!"* Yes this persona keeps you stuck in the loop of Time's control intended for you to 'never' feel like you can do it 'perfectly' to continue to negatively berate yourself.

Dear Alice's, this damage can be undone. A narcissistic person cannot *self-reflect* to be self-aware to empathize with HOW their own behaviors genuinely affect others. Since they are incapable of healthy boundaries, you can choose to free yourself from their unhealthy toxicity successfully! Boundaries, Dear Alice, are imperative. You do not have to choose to continue to wear those façade's you were forced to absorb. You were created UNIQUE, and *fearfully* made! Your confidence and MUCHNESS Dear Alice, can be GENUINE! YOUR MUCHNESS matters and the world need to see it! Those kind hearted gifts created in you are for a reason, I say!

There is another tool a narcissistic abuser uses...provocation of everyone else and calmness. There are some narcissists capable of behaving calmly in situations when another narcissist exhibits rage. However, this calmness is a manipulative tactic to control someone else or used to prove *the narcissist is not the one with the problem*...that *everyone else* is the problem because they are calm when everyone else is upset. I will go more into overt and covert in the second book of the series of '*My Heart My Broken Heart Twisted Wonderland.*'

"I pray FREEDOM over your hearts, minds, emotions, past, present, futures, Dear Alice's in the Name of Jesus Christ! May you all be healed, restored, and made whole to Get Up, Be Raised Up, Grow! May the traumas from your past, the torment of the abuse be released from your spirit, giving place to freedom! May you not be bound mind body spirit to evil that defiles you, and may you FEEL release from what tried to bind you! By the BLOOD of the spotless Lamb of God, may you release the anger, disappointment, envy, chaos, abandonment, rejection, control, responsibility of the abuser, and be mentally, physically, spiritually FREE!"

Blessings, True Alice's and Queens! WALK in the freedom of your authority in peace from within! Bring out your muchness!

Dr. Tia Buchanan, M.A., M.A., M.S., DMin., LPCS, LPC, LAC, NCCA LCCC, NCCA ABCST, EMDRC, ISSA EPFT, ISSA CYI, ISSA CKIC

ABOUT THE AUTHOR

Dr. Tia Buchanan

Dr. Tia Buchanan, a Licensed Professional Counselor, LPC Supervisor, Licensed Addiction Counselor, NCCA Licensed Clinical Christian Counselor, NCCA Certified Sexual Therapist, EMDR Clinician, DCEMin., M.A., M.A, M.S., Certified Play Therapist, Court Involved Therapist, Certified Six-Sigma Black Belt.

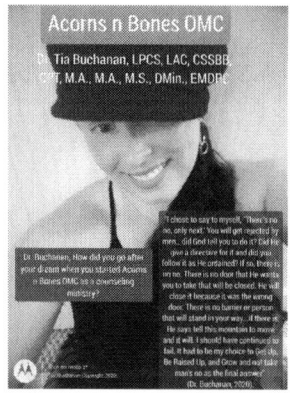

BOOKS BY THIS AUTHOR

My Heart My Broken Heart (Tween, Teen Ages 9+)

Alice is lost and she feels trapped...ALONE within the nightmarish confines of Twisted Wonderland by a narcissistic abuser named Time! She has forgotten who she is. Alice faces the fight of her life against the Jabberwocky...with his claws that bite, his jaws that snatch! She faces off against the Cheshire Cat and even herself.

Alice is stuck within the confines and muck in a world of anthropomorphic creatures who do not understand her...who are all MAD! Feeling heartbroken, lost, and alone, will she give up on herself and succumb to their twisted plots to kill, steal, and destroy her, or will she find the courage to fight her way out and reveal her true self?

My Heart: My Broken Heart reflects diverse feelings of 'madness' of emotional and psychological abuse and is based on characters of Lewis Carroll's "Alice's Adventures in Wonderland," (Carroll, L., 1865) series. The various illustrations throughout this special CHILDREN'S EDITION are a plethora of mixed media from both Lewis Carroll (1865) originals adapted and illustrated to match the emotional states within traumas of psychological physical and emotional abuse. "My Heart My Broken Heart" CHILDREN'S EDITION includes a collection of the authors original digital recreations. You will find many are collages that allow readers to spend a significant amount of time playing 'I spy' to.

What will you discover within the pages of this Twisted Wonderland? Will you discover the Real Alice's way out?
Ages 9 and UP PLUS Tween, Teen, Adults

My Heart My Broken Heart Original

Alice is trapped...in the nightmarish confines of Twisted Wonderland by a narcissistic abuser. My Heart My Broken Heart reflects the coldness and dissonance experienced when you are lost and nothing more than a tool used by a manipulative abuser in an unhealthy, toxic relationship...not only with those she chose and trusted, but with herself. Abuse has many sides of the same coin, and every time it flips, another variable is brought into play. One of the players Alice has forgotten is herself, what tainted destruction she has absorbed...the residual tendrilled effects of seeds planted from the narcissistic abuser. The residual effects of emotional and psychological abuse are serious. These types of abuses escalate to physical abuse and violence. Domestic violence survivors keep secrets of their abuser. Loyalty is a trait they rely on. My Heart: My Broken Heart reflects the diverse experiences of the madness of emotional and psychological abuse, based on "Alice's Adventures in Wonderland," (Carroll, L., 1865). Can Alice escape not only with her life, but with her sanity?
HARDBACK PLUS version includes full color images, plus companion guide.
THIS VERSION TWEEN-ADULT ages.

My Heart My Broken Heart Children's Edition: Paperback

Alice is lost and she feels trapped...ALONE within the nightmarish confines of Twisted Wonderland by a narcissistic abuser named Time! She has forgotten who she is. Alice faces the fight of her life against the Jabberwocky...with his claws that bite, his jaws that snatch! She faces off against the Cheshire Cat and even herself.

Alice is stuck within the confines and muck in a world of anthropomorphic creatures who do not understand her...who are all MAD! Feeling heartbroken, lost, and alone, will she give up on herself and succumb to their twisted plots to kill, steal, and destroy her, or will she find the courage to fight her way out and reveal her true self?

This SPECIAL CHILDREN'S EDITION is dedicated to all children (AND even adults of all ages) to learn there are others who may be experiencing abuse, neglect, bullying, suicidal thoughts, using actions of self-harm, using substances to escape, struggling with behavior issues because of tough stuff going on at home no one knows about...those who exhibit anxiety, depression, irritability with other peer group interactions...you name it from feeling bullied, controlled, or abused. Trauma reactions for adolescents are different in expressions from adults. Adolescents play out thier pains in class, on playgrounds, in private. They act it out...with peers, with teachers, mentors, parents, siblings, themselves. They mimic homelife in ways viewed as behavioral issues through interruptions, distractions, irritability, outbursts, self-harm, bullying others. Those are behaviors and not necessarily ADHD, oppositional defiance, or willful disobedience alone. There is a ROOT. Sometimes children are suffering egregiously because of compounding complex trauma and there is a person in their lives who are (or may be) narcissistically abusing them who pass and skate by in plain sight because of narcissistic glib, charm, and public image protections.

My Heart: My Broken Heart reflects diverse feelings of 'madness' of emotional and psychological abuse and is based on characters of Lewis Carroll's "Alice's Adventures in Wonderland," (Carroll, L., 1865) series. The various illustrations throughout this special CHILDREN'S EDITION are a plethora of mixed media from both Lewis Carroll (1865) originals I adapted and illustrated to match the emotional states within traumas of psychological physical and emotional abuse. "My Heart My Broken Heart" CHILDREN'S EDITION includes a collection of my original digital recreations. You will find many are collages that allow readers to spend a significant amount of time playing 'I spy' to. What will you discover within the pages of this Twisted Wonderland? Will you discover the Real Alice's way out?

Ages 9 and up suggested, TWEEN, TEEN ADULTS ENJOY the seek and find FULL COLOR originally adapted illustrations!

My Heart My Broken Heart Journal The Trap ((Alice In Wonderland) My Heart My Broken Heart In Twisted Wonderland's) Paperback

Teachers, Mentors, Parents, Caregivers, Therapists, parents...you may use this journal with your teens, adolescents, kids at age 2 and up, and yourselves!

This is a companion journal to the "My Heart My Broken Heart" illustrated series, Chapter Six, 'The Trap,' and is for adults and adolescents of all ages. As a clinician for more than 12 years, in therapy, I have used logs, questionnaires, journals, and other writing forms to help my people heal from stresses and traumas. This journal is for any use. If you choose to use this journal with "My Heart My Broken Heart," enlightenment can occur through writing compares and free exploration in psychodynamic psychotherapies. Nothing is a wrong answer in this exploration. You may write, scribble, draw emotions. For some, writing about trauma triggers distress and physical and emotional arousal will work through distress and for some, drawing, scribbling, doodling, movement of the pen or pencil on paper in any way is also therapeutic without using words. This journal is for ages 2 and UP!

My Heart My Broken Heart Journal: Tunnel Of Nightmares ((Alice In Wonderland) My Heart My Broken Heart In Twisted Wonderland's) Paperback

Teachers, Mentors, Parents, Caregivers, Therapists, parents...you may use this journal with your teens, adolescents, kids at age 2 and up, and yourselves!

This is a companion journal to the "My Heart My Broken Heart" illustrated series, Chapter Five, 'Jabberwocky,' with the illustration "Tunnel of Nightmares" (Buchanan, 2022), and is for adults and adolescents of all ages. As a clinician for more than 12 years, in therapy, I have used logs, questionnaires, journals, and other writing forms to help my people heal from stresses and traumas.

This journal is for any use. If you choose to use this journal with "My Heart My Broken Heart," enlightenment can occur through writing compares and free exploration in psychodynamic psychotherapies. Nothing is a wrong answer in this exploration. You may write, scribble, draw emotions. For some, writing about trauma triggers distress and physical and emotional arousal will work through distress and for some, drawing, scribbling, doodling, movement of the pen or pencil on paper in any way is also therapeutic without using words. This journal is for ages 2 and UP!

My Heart My Broken Heart Journal Jabberwocky ((Alice In Wonderland) My Heart My Broken Heart In Twisted Wonderland's) Paperback

Teachers, Mentors, Parents, Caregivers, Therapists, parents...you may use this journal with your teens, adolescents, kids at age 2 and up, and yourselves!

This is a companion journal to the "My Heart My Broken Heart" illustrated series, Chapter Five, 'Jabberwocky,' and is for adults and adolescents of all ages. As a clinician for more than 12 years, in therapy, I have used logs, questionnaires, journals, and other writing forms to help my people heal from stresses and traumas.

This journal is for any use. If you choose to use this journal with "My Heart My Broken Heart," enlightenment can occur through writing compares and free exploration in psychodynamic psychotherapies. Nothing is a wrong answer in this exploration. You may write, scribble, draw emotions. For some, writing about trauma triggers distress and physical and emotional arousal will work through distress and for some, drawing, scribbling, doodling,

movement of the pen or pencil on paper in any way is also therapeutic without using words. This journal is for ages 2 and UP!

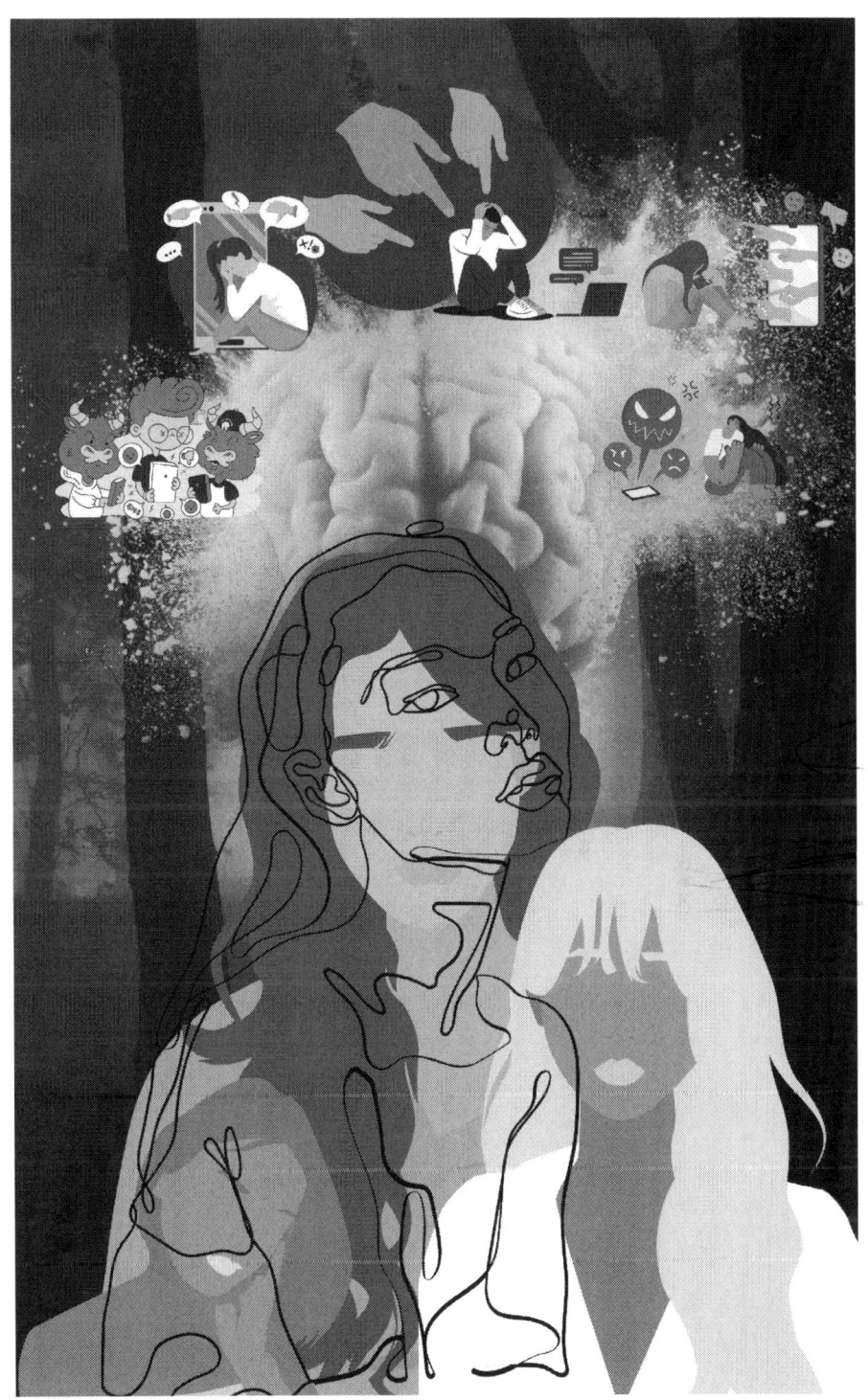

Made in the USA
Columbia, SC
13 April 2022

58874274R00057